A Handbook of
Gastroesophageal Reflux Disease

A Handbook of
Gastroesophageal Reflux Disease

Vinod Kumar Nigam
MBBS MS FICS FIAGES
Principal Consultant
(General and Minimal Access Surgery and GI Endoscopy)
Max Hospital
Gurugram, Haryana, India

Siddharth Nigam
MBBS MS (General Surgery)
Senior Consultant
(General and Minimal Access Surgery)
Max Hospital
Gurugram, Haryana, India

Foreword
Vivek Raj

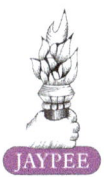

JAYPEE BROTHERS MEDICAL PUBLISHERS
The Health Sciences Publisher
New Delhi | London

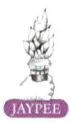
Jaypee Brothers Medical Publishers (P) Ltd

Headquarters
Jaypee Brothers Medical Publishers (P) Ltd
EMCA House, 23/23-B
Ansari Road, Daryaganj
New Delhi 110 002, India
Landline: +91-11-23272143, +91-11-23272703
+91-11-23282021, +91-11-23245672
Email: jaypee@jaypeebrothers.com

Corporate Office
Jaypee Brothers Medical Publishers (P) Ltd
4838/24, Ansari Road, Daryaganj
New Delhi 110 002, India
Phone: +91-11-43574357
Fax: +91-11-43574314
Email: jaypee@jaypeebrothers.com

Overseas Office
JP Medical Ltd
83 Victoria Street, London
SW1H 0HW (UK)
Phone: +44 20 3170 8910
Email: info@jpmedpub.com

EU GPSR Authorised Representative
Logos Europe, 9 rue Nicolas Poussin
17000, La Rochelle, France
Phone: +33 (0) 6 67 93 73 78
E-mail: Contact@logoseurope.eu

Website: www.jaypeebrothers.com
Website: www.jaypeedigital.com

© 2024, Jaypee Brothers Medical Publishers

The views and opinions expressed in this book are solely those of the original contributor(s)/author(s) and do not necessarily represent those of editor(s) or publisher of the book.

All rights reserved. No part of this publication may be reproduced, stored or transmitted in any form or by any means, electronic, mechanical, photocopying, recording or otherwise, without the prior permission in writing of the publishers.

All brand names and product names used in this book are trade names, service marks, trademarks or registered trademarks of their respective owners. The publisher is not associated with any product or vendor mentioned in this book.

Medical knowledge and practice change constantly. This book is designed to provide accurate, authoritative information about the subject matter in question. However, readers are advised to check the most current information available on procedures included and check information from the manufacturer of each product to be administered, to verify the recommended dose, formula, method and duration of administration, adverse effects and contra-indications. It is the responsibility of the practitioner to take all appropriate safety precautions. Neither the publisher nor the author(s)/editor(s) assume any liability for any injury and/or damage to persons or property arising from or related to use of material in this book.

This book is sold on the understanding that the publisher is not engaged in providing professional medical services. If such advice or services are required, the services of a competent medical professional should be sought.

Every effort has been made where necessary to contact holders of copyright to obtain permission to reproduce copyright material. If any have been inadvertently overlooked, the publisher will be pleased to make the necessary arrangements at the first opportunity.

Inquiries for bulk sales may be solicited at: jaypee@jaypeebrothers.com

A Handbook of Gastroesophageal Reflux Disease

First Edition: 2024

ISBN: 978-93-5696-944-5

Dedicated to

Late Sh KB Nigam (Father of author and Grandfather of co-author)
Late Smt CK Nigam (Mother of author and Grandmother of co-author)
Mrs Kumud Nigam (Wife of author and Mother of co-author)
for their untiring support and encouragement throughout the journey
and
All our patients.

Vinod Kumar Nigam
Siddharth Nigam

Foreword

Gastroesophageal reflux disease (GERD) is one of the most common diseases in the world. In India, *Gas, Acidity, Bloating,* and *Dyspepsia* are some of the most common symptoms that patients consult their doctor for. Despite being one of the most common conditions which affects almost half the population at some point in their lives and about 10% of population, on a very frequent basis, the knowledge of the pathophysiology, management principles, drug management, surgical options, etc. is poorly understood by many doctors. With the advent of proton-pump inhibitors and good promotility agents, management of GERD has become much easier. However, in the process of simplifying treatment, one needs to remember the essential role of lifestyle modification, and where indicated, surgery.

Vinod Kumar Nigam and Sidharth Nigam have written a fantastic handbook in a very simple and easy-to-understand format. They have illustrated the book with diagrams and images which make it very easy-to-understand the complexities of anatomy, physiology, and management principles of GERD.

Vinod Kumar Nigam is a very experienced Surgeon. He is currently Principal Consultant (General and Minimal Access Surgery and GI Endoscopy), Max Hospital, Gurugram, Haryana, India. He trained in India and Scotland and has an illustrious career spanning more than 4 decades. He has not only written textbooks for surgery including *Essentials of Abdominal wall Hernias* but also books on *History of Medicine and Spiritual Aspects of Medicine*. His book *40 Minutes with God* is a bestseller. His other books include *Science, Faith, and Medicine,* and *Do you Want to Live Long and Healthy*. Besides the books, he has numerous national and international publications. Teaching is his passion.

Siddharth Nigam, the Co-Author of this handbook, is a highly accomplished Surgeon with more than a decade of experience. He is currently Senior Consultant (General and Minimal Access Surgery), Max Hospital, Gurugram, Haryana, India. He is also a prolific Writer and has co-authored 3 books including *40 Minutes with God, An Introduction to History of Medicine,* and *Essentials of Abdominal Wall Hernia*. He has also invented a surgical technique for abdominal hernia—NICH.

In this day of overload of information and many sources of information, it is wonderful to see a handbook which is comprehensive, and yet easy to understand. The handbook will be extremely useful for general physicians, young gastroenterologists, and surgeons alike. It is a breath of fresh air. I wish Drs Nigam all success.

Vivek Raj
MD FRCP
Principal Director and Head of Department
Center for Gastroenterology
Hepatology and Endoscopy
Max Superspeciality Hospital
Saket, New Delhi
Max Hospital, Gurugram
Haryana, India

Preface

The practice of gastroenterology requires sufficient knowledge of anatomy and physiology of the upper gastrointestinal tract. Technological development in gastroenterology is tremendous, which is phenomenal. Earlier, the etiology of gastritis and gastric duodenal ulcers was considered to be due to unhealthy lifestyle such as smoking and consuming spicy food, alcohol, and painkillers, but now the scenario has changed completely after identification of *Helicobacter pylori* bacteria. It has now been proven that these problems are caused by *H. pylori* infection and are completely treatable. This research advancement has made lives of million patients' pain-free and comfortable. The development of ulcer-healing medicines and *H. pylori*-eradicating medicines has made the incidence of gastric and duodenal ulcers and cancer of stomach significantly low. H_2-receptor antagonist and proton-pump inhibitors have made lives very comfortable and have reduced the complications arising from these problems.

Gastroesophageal reflux disease (GERD) is a very common problem and it used to give discomfort and suffering up to such a degree that operative management was required commonly. Nissen's fundoplication was most commonly used compared to nowadays. It all happened due to very effective and potent drugs.

This book deals with one of the most common problems of gastroenterology, GERD and *H. pylori* gastritis. This book has visual details in the form of photographs and diagrams in relation to GERD which makes a student understand the subject better, quickly, and clearly without wasting much time. The line diagrams are made to explain the problems easily. This book is a handbook for technicians and MBBS students also. The book is helpful to young doctors, physicians and surgeons who are longing to know more about GERD.

Chapter on *Controversies, Arguments and Discussions* is there to understand different views and to follow the overall accepted procedures and to know the pros and cons of various ways of dealing with a situation. Recent advancements and modern trends make the reader aware of what is recent and what is obsolete. Pharmacology of drugs used in GERD will be helpful to the students. The chapter on *Frequently Asked Questions* by the patients is important from the patient's point of view as this book is also a general book for persons suffering with GERD.

Vinod Kumar Nigam
Siddharth Nigam

Acknowledgments

We are thankful to all our colleagues who helped us by providing valuable information, suggestions, and photographs used in this book. We thank Dr Kunal Nigam, an ENT Surgeon, for helping us to write anatomy and other basic sciences. Dr Madhur Arora, a Critical Care Consultant, helped us by drawing beautiful line diagrams and searching medical literature and references. Dr Charvi Chawla, deserves thanks for proofreading and suggestions.

Mrs Kumud Nigam, for allowing me to take as much time as required from personal life to devote to writing this book without any complaints. She also did an excellent job of proofreading of the book. Mr Vipin Sharma earns our thanks and gratitude for typing and computer related work.

We especially appreciate the constant support and encouragement of Shri Jitendar P Vij (Group Chairman) and Mr Ankit Vij (Managing Director) of M/s Jaypee Brothers Medical Publishers (P) Ltd, New Delhi, India, in publishing the book and also their associates, particularly Ms Chetna Malhotra (Senior Director—Professional Publishing, Marketing, and Business Development) and Ms Pragati Singh (Development Editor) who have been prompt, efficient, and most helpful.

Vinod Kumar Nigam
Siddharth Nigam

Contents

1. Introduction 1
2. Surgical Anatomy of Esophagus, Gastroesophageal Junction, and Lower Esophageal Sphincter 5
3. Physiology of Esophagus, Gastroesophageal Junction, and Lower Esophageal Sphincter 16
4. Histology of Esophagus 23
5. Epidemiology of Gastroesophageal Reflux Disease 26
6. Etiology of Gastroesophageal Reflux Disease 28
7. Pathophysiology of Gastroesophageal Reflux Disease 31
8. Clinical Features of Gastroesophageal Reflux Disease 34
9. Diagnosis of Gastroesophageal Reflux Disease 50
10. Differential Diagnosis of Gastroesophageal Reflux Disease 54
11. Complications of Gastroesophageal Reflux Disease 63
12. Prognosis 66
13. Management of Gastroesophageal Reflux Disease 67
14. Barrett's Esophagus 75
15. Hiatus Hernia 82
16. *Helicobacter pylori* Infection 85
17. Recent Advancements and Modern Trends in Gastroesophageal Reflux Disease 88
18. Pharmacology of Drugs Used in Gastroesophageal Reflux Disease 89
19. What Questions Patient may Ask about Gastroesophageal Reflux Disease 91
20. Some Interesting Cases of Gastroesophageal Reflux Disease 97

Abbreviations *119*
Multiple Choice Questions and True/False *120*
Index *123*

CHAPTER 1

Introduction

Heartache makes for good poetry, heartburn not so much.
—S Tarr

Gastroesophageal reflux disease (GERD) is a global gastrointestinal problem. GERD happens when your stomach contents comeback up into your esophagus also called backwash (acid reflux). GERD if occurs recurrently for long then it can lead to complications.[1]

The Montreal definition and classification of GERD is an excellent well-constructed guideline, compiled by world authorities on the subject, after exhaustive consultation. The success of any guidelines is to achieve wide recognition and ensure uniformity in approach.[2]

GERD was defined as a condition that develops when the reflux of stomach contents causes troublesome symptoms and/or complications. Most of us will suffer with GERD sometime in our lives. Approximately half of all adults will report reflux symptoms at sometimes.[3] Most of us can manage GERD with lifestyle changes, around only a small percentage of persons do not get relief from these nonsurgical treatments, they require surgical treatment such as Nissen's fundoplication.

It is right to start treatment of GERD such as PPIs if symptoms are same as of classification symptoms of GERD. If the long-standing suspected cases of GERD do not respond to empirical therapy or there are alarming symptoms such as dysphagia, odynophagia, weight loss or there is suspicion of complications such as Barrett's esophagus, early upper gastrointestinal endoscopy is advised.

Severity of GERD symptoms is not directly proportional to the incidence of complications of GERD.

Upper gastrointestinal endoscopy with biopsy is the gold standard to diagnose the complications of GERD such as Berrett's esophagus and adenocarcinoma of esophagus even in very early stage. There is no need of biopsy in normal looking esophageal mucosa on endoscopy.

Barium studies cannot be compared with endoscopy for diagnosis of complications of GERD. Endoscopy has surpassed barium studies due to its advantages over barium studies.

Foods that relax lower esophageal sphincter (LES) and lead to reflux are chocolates, peppermint, coffee, smoking, alcohol, onions, and garlic. The sensitivity of these food items leading to or worsening of GERD symptoms is also related to biological individuality.

Usually, the persons with off and on reflux symptoms use over-the-counter (OTC) medicines and antacids and get relief and so they do not require continuous proton pump inhibitor (PPI) treatment. There may be a role of some placebo effect also in such cases. H_2-receptor antagonists and PPIs are generally quite competent in dealing with problems of GERD and are advised to be used for at least 2 weeks.

The GERD is actually an acronym and not an abbreviation. GERD is a common problem and large number of people are diagnosed with GERD annually in India alone. A big percentage of GERD patients are getting relief with lifestyle changes and OTC medicines. Some require specific treatment and very few require surgical treatment. The prevalence of GERD among global population reminds of a quote, by Hippocrates "Death sits in the bowels. All disease begins in the gut". He was not far from the truth. Gut bacteria and gut mucosal inflammation cause many common health problems of today including GERD, as lining of esophagus gets irritated by acid from stomach leading to inflammation and ulcerations. GERD is a very common digestive disorder worldwide with an estimated prevalence of 18.1–27.8% in North America.[4]

Gastroesophageal reflux disease has esophageal and extraesophageal symptoms. Classical esophageal symptoms are usually heart burns and regurgitation. The patients who show presence of classical GERD symptoms should be treated with empirical therapy. Patients who show signs of GERD complication or other illness or who do not respond to therapy should be considered for further diagnostic testing.[5] Most of the persons suffering with GERD have frequent heartburn; even some have it daily and regularly. This is a very annoying and disturbing feeling. As the name of the problem is GERD, it is self-explanatory that acid of the stomach with gastric contents refluxly move backward and enter esophagus. If stomach content persistently and regularly flows up into the esophagus, resulting in symptoms and/or complications.[6] The backflow of gastric contents and acid is due to patulous, loose or incompetent LES, or gastroesophageal junction. Backflow of gastric contents into esophagus is not an abnormal feature as it occurs occasionally, it is also called acid reflux, when you overeat. When it is associated with symptoms such as retrosternal burning, bitter taste, chest pain, and nausea then it is called GERD **(Figs. 1A and B)**.

When we eat food, it goes from mouth to the pharynx and then to the esophagus or food pipe. Esophagus has a muscle sphincter or a

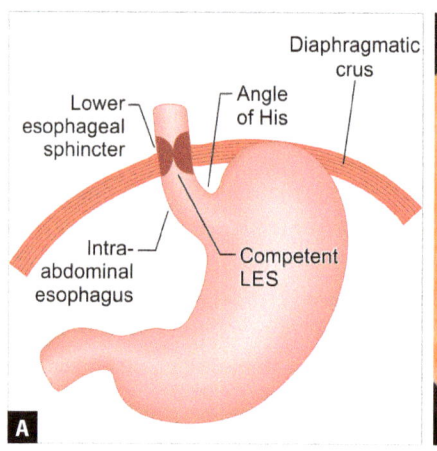
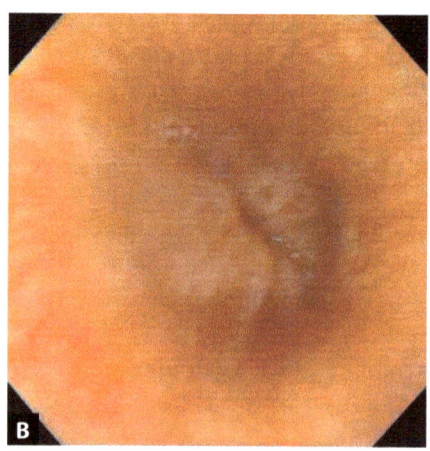

Figs. 1A and B: Competent lower esophageal sphincter in a normal individual.

ring called lower esophageal sphincter (LES) which opens when food reaches at lower end of esophagus and then allows food to enter the stomach, then LES contracts and closes the esophagogastric junction so that when churning of food happens in the stomach the food and acid cannot leak out to esophagus but sometimes even in a normal person this LES does not close properly and completely so the acid with gastric contents flows back to the esophagus. It happens occasionally and especially after a big meal. It is taken as a normal phenomenon. When this occurs frequently due to incompetent LES **(Figs. 2A and B)** and with symptoms, then it is called GERD. The symptoms of GERD may be present with or without esophageal mucosal injury.

It is found in various researches that almost half of the patients of gastric reflux suffer with esophagitis. Most common symptoms of GERD are heartburn and pain in epigastrium **(Figs. 3A and B)**.

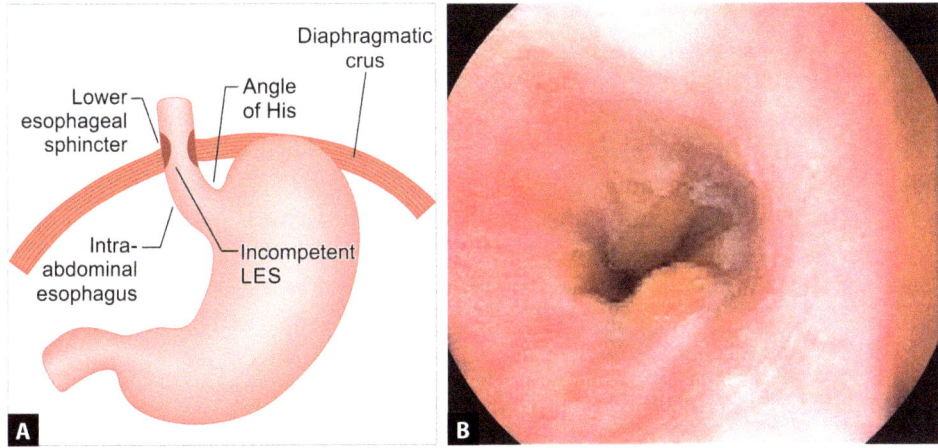

Figs. 2A and B: Incompetent LES in GERD.
(GERD: gastroesophageal reflux disease; LES: lower esophageal sphincter)

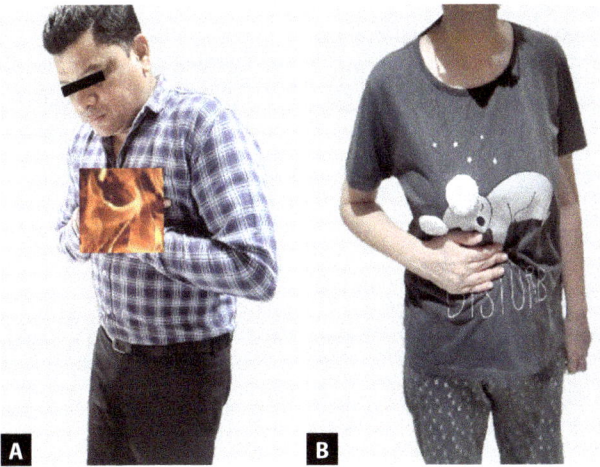

Figs. 3A and B: (A) Fire in chest—heartburn; (B) Pain in epigastrium in gastroesophageal reflux disease.

You must consult a physician when you have following symptoms:
- Constant or regular chest pain
- Painful swallowing
- Difficulty in swallowing
- Persistent vomiting
- Blood in vomit
- Black tarry stools

It is called GERD in USA and GORD in UK. GERD can cause troublesome symptoms and have a significant impact on quality of life.[7]

Guidelines for the diagnosis and treatment of GERD were published by American College of Gastroenterology in 1995 and updated in 1999.[8,9]

These and other guidelines undergo periodic review. GERD develops mucosal damage by gastric refluxate containing acid which is corrosive and this is the main reason for symptoms and complications.

REFERENCES

1. Vakil N, Van Zanten SV, Kahrilas P, Dent J, Jones R; Global Consensus Group. The Montreal Definition and Classification of Gastroesophageal Reflux Disease: a global evidence-based consensus. Am J Gastroenterol. 2006;101:1900-20.
2. Schnieder HR. Gastro-oesophageal reflux disease: the Montreal Definition and Classification. SA Fam Pract. 2007;49(1):19-26.
3. Locke GR 3rd, Talley NJ, Fett SL, Zinsmeister AR, Melton LJ 3rd. Prevalence and clinical spectrum of gastroesophageal reflux: a population-based study in Olmsted County, Minnesota. Gastroentrology. 1997;112:1448-56.
4. El-Serag HB, Sweet S, Winchester CC, Dent J. Update on the epidemiology of gastroesophageal reflux disease: a systematic review. Gut. 2014;63:871-80.
5. DoVault KR, Castelf DO. Updated guidelines for the diagnosis and treatment of gastroesophageal reflux disease. Am J Gastroenterol. 2005;100(1):190-200.
6. Kahrilas PJ, Shaheen NJ, Vaezi MF. American Gastrological Association Institute Technical Review on the Management of Gastroesophageal Reflux Disease. Gastroenterology. 2008;135(4):1392-413.
7. Jack J, Becher A, Mulligan C, Johson DA. Systemic review: The burden of disruptive gastroesophageal reflux disease on health-related quality of life. Aliment Pharmacol Ther. 2012;35:1257-66.
8. De Vault KR, Castell DO. Guidelines for the diagnoses and treatment of gastroesophageal reflux disease. Arch Inrn Med. 1995;155:2165-73.
9. De Vault KR, Castell DO. Updated guidelines for the diagnosis and treatment of gastroesophageal reflux disease. Am J Gastroenterol. 1999;94:1434-42.

CHAPTER 2

Surgical Anatomy of Esophagus, Gastroesophageal Junction, and Lower Esophageal Sphincter

*"Remember that your patient is a human being like yourself,
Your knowledge of anatomy may save his or her life"*

–Richard S Snell

DEVELOPMENT

When organs start appearing in the fetus, the gut develops by folding patterns. During development, the foregut differentiates into the trachea, lungs, and esophagus.[1,2] At approximately 6th week of development, the circular and longitudinal muscular layers begin to form, and ganglion cells of myenteric plexus appear. Moving into week 7, cells of mesoderm originate and proliferate into the submucous layer forming the eventual blood supply to the esophagus. The muscular layers, which began in week 6, are completed by the 9th week.[3] Initially, the esophagus is very short but it elongates rapidly with the growth of fetus. The epithelium of the esophagus proliferates and almost obliterates the lumen but recanalization occurs at a later age. The respiratory system arises as the laryngotracheal diverticulum from the primitive pharynx **(Fig. 1)**. It grows gradually and becomes separated. Congenital anomalies may arise if there is interference with the normal development of the trachea and esophagus.[4]

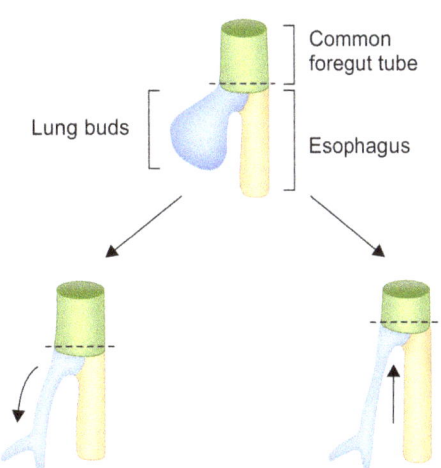

Fig. 1: Development of esophagus and respiratory system.

ANATOMY OF ESOPHAGUS

Esophagus is a muscular tube which basically functions as a pathway to transfer the food from pharynx to the stomach. When there is no food in esophagus, it remains empty and deflated with 2–3 cm diameter. Esophagus can distend and stretch to some degree (>2–3 cm) to accommodate a bigger bolus of food.

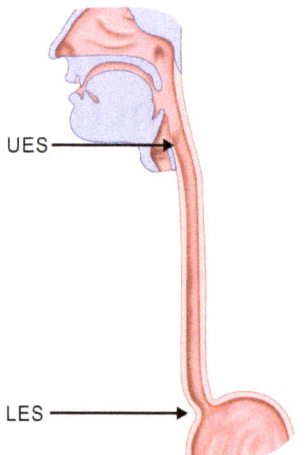

Fig. 2: Upper and lower esophageal sphincters.

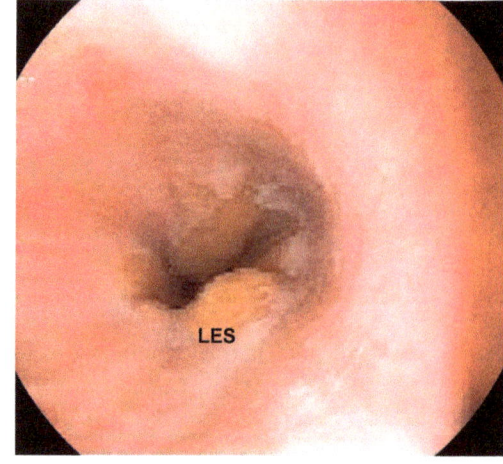

Fig. 4: Lower esophageal sphincter (LES).

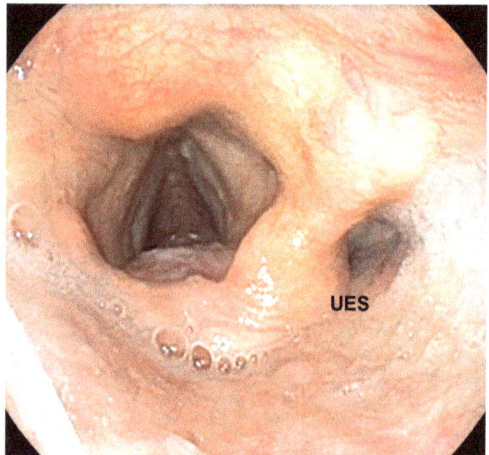

Fig. 3: Upper esophageal sphincter (UES).

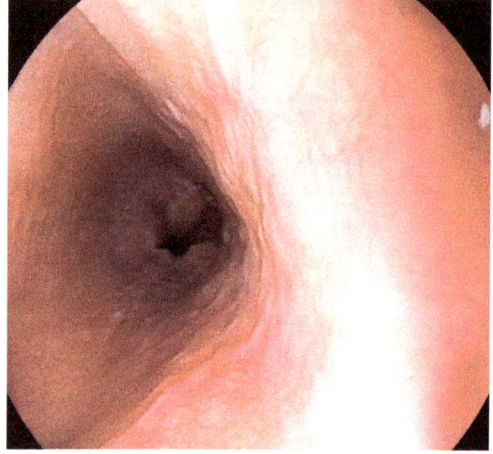

Fig. 5: Normal esophagus, cervical, thoracic, and abdominal.

Esophagus in adult is approximately 25 cm long. It starts from cricoid cartilage (C6 vertebra) and ends at esophagogastric junction (T11 vertebra). Dilatation of esophagus, Upper esophageal sphincter (UES) and lower esophageal sphincter (LES) allows even a big bolus of food **(Figs. 2 to 4)**.

During its course, the esophagus encounters three anatomic constrictions:[5]
1. At the level of the cricopharyngeus muscle
2. As it travels posterior to the aortic arch/ left mainstem bronchus, and
3. At the level of esophageal hiatus of the diaphragm. These areas of constriction are considered the most frequent sites for a foreign body or food impaction to occur.

PARTS OF ESOPHAGUS

Esophagus has three parts **(Fig. 5)**:
1. Cervical esophagus
2. Thoracic esophagus
3. Abdominal esophagus

Cervical Esophagus

It is 5–6 cm long. Cervical esophagus travels between lower border of cricoid cartilage and the thoracic inlet. Important feature of cervical esophagus is that the recurrent laryngeal nerve travels on each side in a space between esophagus and trachea **(Fig. 7C)**.

Thoracic Esophagus

It is present in superior and posterior mediastinum between trachea and vertebral column **(Fig. 6)** and in the posterior mediastinum it comes anterior to aorta. It extends from thoracic inlet to the diaphragm **(Fig. 7B)**

Abdominal Esophagus

It is about 2.5 cm in length and lies on the posterior surface of left lobe of liver. It is covered by peritoneum on its front and left side **(Fig. 7A)**.

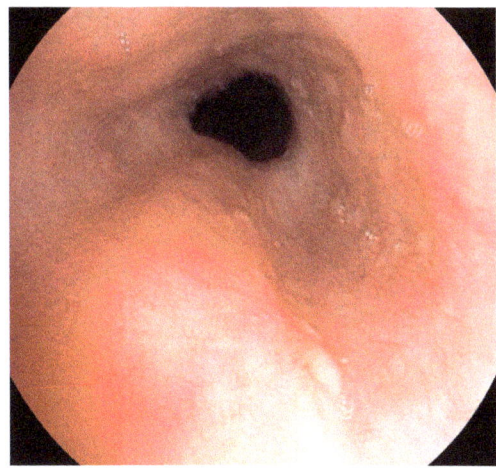

Fig. 6: Indentation of vertebral column in normal esophagus.

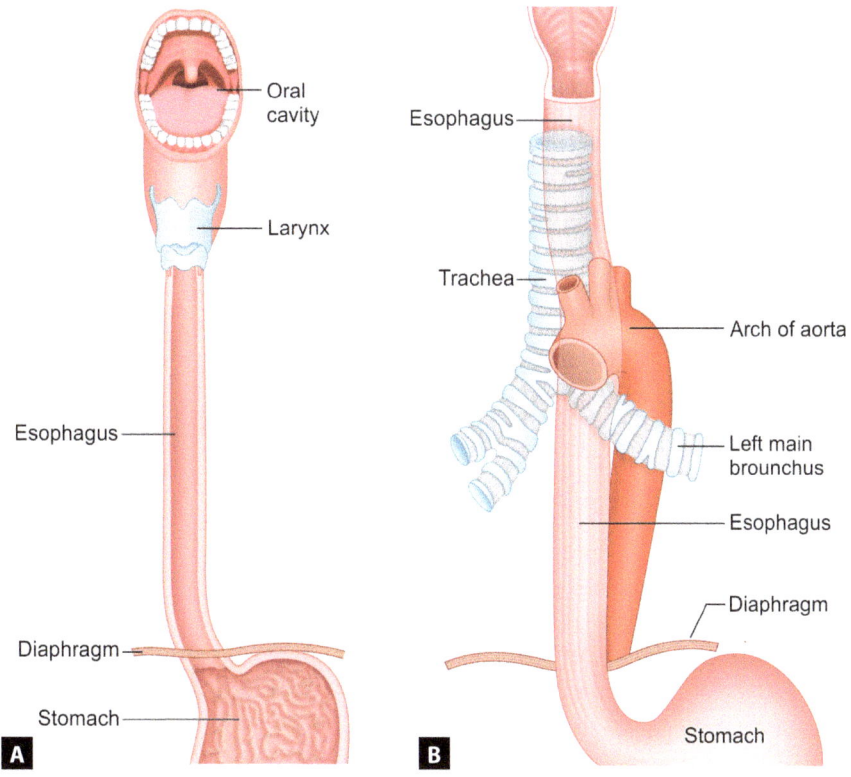

Figs. 7A and B

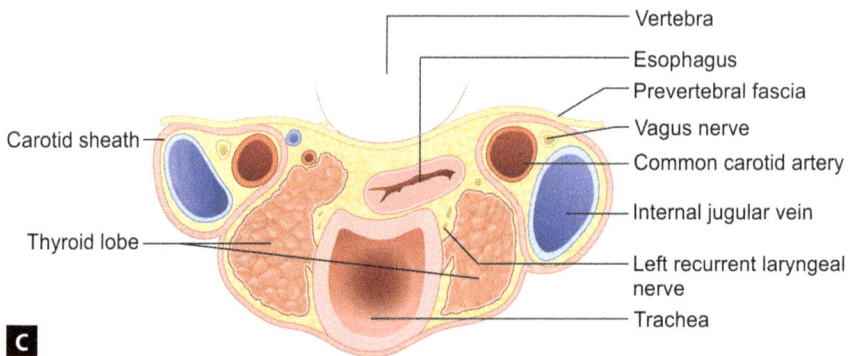

Figs. 7A to C: (A and B) Esophagus in its course and (C) the cervical esophagus on cross-section.

Relations of Abdominal Esophagus

It lies at the level of 11th and 12th thoracic vertebrae **(Fig. 8)**.

- *Anterior:*
  - Posterior surface of left lobe of liver
  - Left vagus nerve
  - Esophageal plexus
- *Posterior:*
  - Crura of diaphragm
  - Aorta
  - Left inferior phrenic artery
- *Right:* The caudate lobe of liver
- *Left:* Gastroesophageal or esophagogastric junction

The function of median arcuate ligament is like a barrier. It is a tough band of muscle fibers, 1–3 mm wide. It is the condensation of fibers of medial crus of the diaphragm **(Fig. 9)**.

GASTROESOPHAGEAL JUNCTION

It is the site where esophagus meets stomach. It is not a well-marked area. Gastroesophageal junction (GEJ) acts as a sphincter and it is a complex sphincter. GEJ has two parts:
1. Extrinsic or external part—diaphragmatic part
2. Intrinsic or internal part—LES

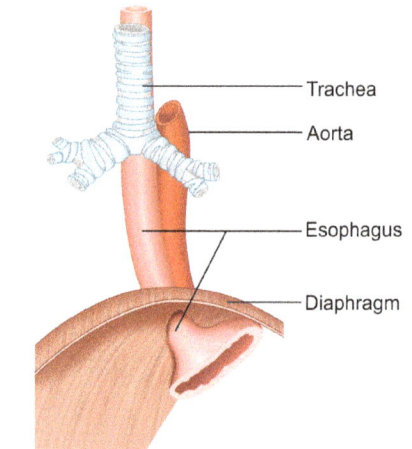

Fig. 8: Thoracic and abdominal parts of esophagus.

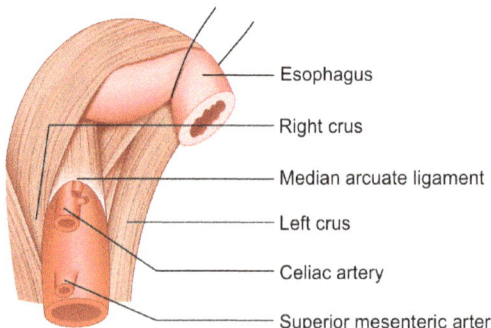

Fig. 9: Esophagus in relation to right and left crura of diaphragm.

So GEJ has both a diaphragmatic element, skeletal muscle and LES, smooth muscle.

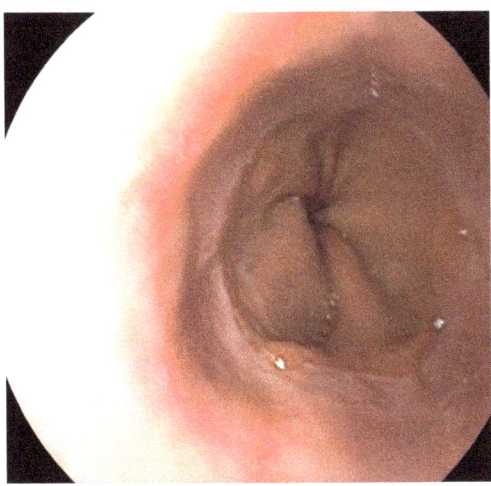

Fig. 10: Intrinsic or internal gastroesophageal junction.

Extrinsic or External Junction

It lies in the abdomen below the diaphragm.

Intrinsic or Internal Junction

The histological junction between esophagus and stomach is marked by an irregular boundary between stratified squamous epithelium of esophagus and gastric simple columnar epithelium.

External and internal junctions do not coincide with each other as the mucosa level changes due to very loose submucosal connective tissue **(Fig. 10)**.

LOWER ESOPHAGEAL SPHINCTER

Lower esophageal sphincter consists of muscle fibers. It has two components:
1. Extrinsic part is formed by diaphragmatic crurae and phrenoesophageal ligament.
2. *Intrinsic part:* It is made of esophageal muscle fibers which are under neurohormonal force. Size of esophageal sphincter increases gradually after birth and LES matures at approximately 2 years of age.

LES is weakened and relaxed by:
- Alcohol
- Smoking
- Caffeine
- Chocolate
- Drugs—blood pressure medications
- Obesity
- Overeating
- Fatty foods
- Spicy foods
- Tomato based foods
- Citrus fruits
- Pregnancy

Lower esophageal sphincter is made up of smooth muscles and then sphincter remains contracted except during swallowing. It is contracted due to both myogenic (muscular) and neurogenic (nerve) factors. The diaphragmatic sphincter muscle is made up of skeletal muscle fibers. The myogenic contraction by gastrointestinal smooth muscle contracts and relaxes.

As previously discussed, the LES is comprised of an intrinsic and an extrinsic component. Any malfunction in either of these components can lead to pathologies such as gastroesophageal reflux disease (GERD) with its associated symptoms and mucosal changes. Additionally, a structurally defective LES and a hiatus hernia are important factors in the pathogenesis of reflux disease.[6]

The LES is innervated by both parasympathetic (vagus) and sympathetic (splanchnic) nerves.

The sphincter at the lower end of esophagus is helped by several other structures—the angle (of His) at which the esophagus enters the stomach, the pinchcock action of the diaphragm, a plug of loose esophageal mucosa (mucosal rosette), the phrenoesophageal membrane, and the sling of oblique fibers of the gastric musculature.[7]

Transient Lower Esophageal Sphincter Relaxation

Lower esophageal sphincter relaxations (LESRs) are one of the most common processes of causing GERD even when the LES pressure is normal. During swallowing process, LESR occurs for <10 seconds. LESRs is a normal mechanism in healthy persons with normal LES. It is a dominant phenomenon in GERD as in it, LESRs occur too frequently and for longer periods (>10 seconds). Most GERD attacks occur during LESRs. LESRs are not associated with swallowing phenomenon.

- *Intrinsic component of LES:* Esophageal smooth muscle fiber
- *Extrinsic component of LES:*
  - Diaphragmatic crura
  - Phrenoesophageal ligament

Right Crus of Diaphragm

Esophageal hiatus of diaphragm is located in right crus of diaphragm. LES is made up of smooth muscles. It is 2-4 cm in size. LES is fixed to esophageal hiatus of diaphragm by phrenoesophageal ligament which inserts at lower esophagus. LES is a high-pressure zone. At rest, the LES is in a state of contraction. During swallowing of food, it relaxes and opens up to allow food to pass into stomach.

The right crus of diaphragm causes extrinsic squeeze to the intrinsic LES. This requires approximately 10 mm Hg pressure to LES.

Phrenoesophageal Ligament *(Fig. 11)*

This so-called ligament consists of following structures:
- Pleura
- Subpleural fascia (endothoracic)
- Phrenoesophageal fascia of Laimer
- Transversalis (endoabdominal subdiaphragmatic) fascia
- Peritoneum

Phrenoesophageal ligament acts as a seal around esophagus which is airtight. The seal must be strong enough to resist abdominal pressure that tends to push the stomach into the thorax and flexible enough to give with the pressure changes incidental to the breathing and the movement incidental to swallowing. The first and last of these elements provide

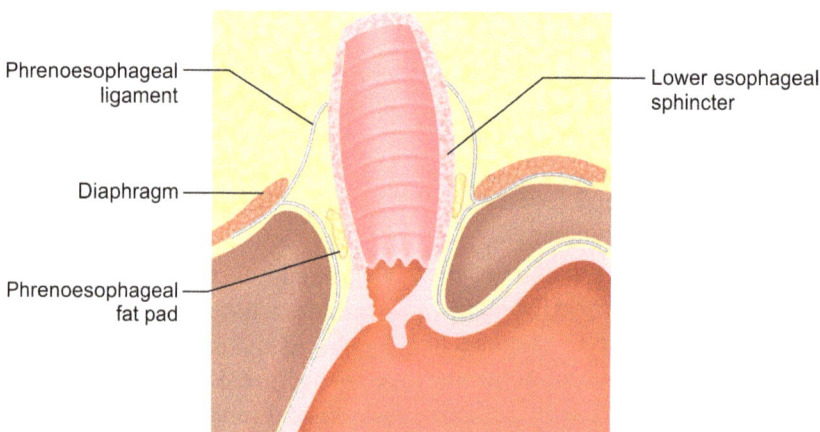

Fig. 11: Gastroesophageal junction and phrenoesophageal ligament.

the requirement for airtightness; the middle three provide flexibility and strength. The ligament exists in infants, is attenuated in adults, and does not exist in adult patients with hiatus hernia.[8]

Note: Because the esophageal neuroanatomic pathways overlap with those of the heart and respiratory system, in clinical practice it may be difficult to discern the organ of origin for some chest pain syndromes.
—Mark Feldman et al. Sleisenger and Fordtran's book "Gastrointestinal and Liver Disease" (10th Edition).

Blood Supply of Esophagus *(Fig. 12)*

The blood supply of the esophagus is from three directions:
1. The upper part is supplied by branches of interior thyroid artery.
2. The main part of esophagus is supplied by esophageal branches of aorta.
3. Lower part of esophagus is supplied by the branches of:
   - Gastric arteries
   - Inferior phrenic artery

Note: The esophageal branches of aorta supplying the main part of the esophagus are very tender, slender, and delicate so they can be damaged by rough handling of esophagus during operation and can cause damage to that part of the esophagus.

Venous Drainage of Esophagus *(Fig. 13)*

The blood from esophagus is drained into three directions as follows:
1. Cervical esophagus veins drain into inferior thyroid vein leading to the brachiocephalic veins.
2. Thoracic esophagus veins drain:
   - On right side into superior vena cava through azygos system
   - On left side veins drain into brachiocephalic vein through left hemiazygos system
3. Veins from esophagogastric junction drain into:
   - Coronary veins
   - Splenic veins
   - Retroperitoneal veins
   - Inferior phrenic vein

These veins ultimately drain into portal and caval systems.

Lymphatic Drainage of Esophagus

Lymphatics of esophagus lie in the submucosa and here they run up and down. They penetrate muscle layer of esophagus and reach to the outer surface of esophagus. There are three main drainage systems of lymphatics of esophagus:
1. Lymphatics from upper one-third of esophagus drain into deep cervical lymph nodes and then lymph goes to thoracic duct.
2. Lymphatics from middle one-third of esophagus drain into superior and posterior mediastinal lymph nodes.

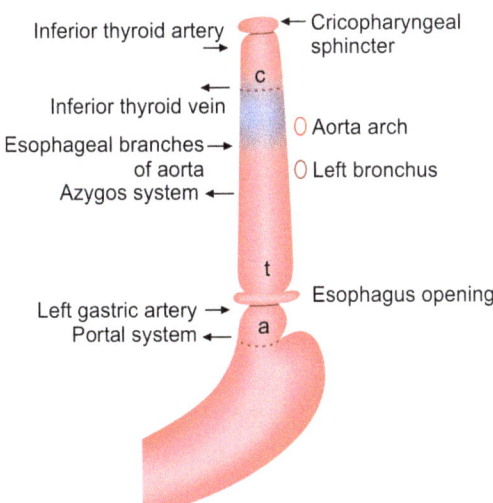

Fig. 12: Blood supply of esophagus.

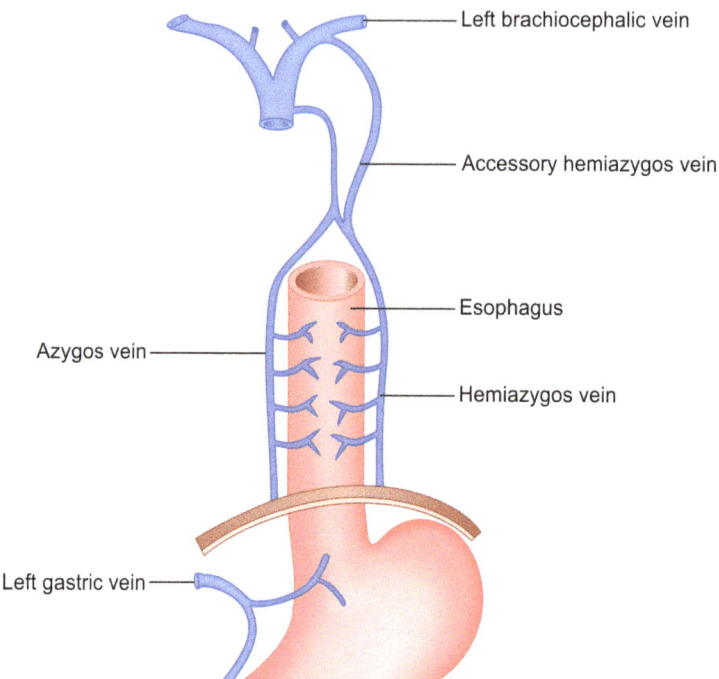

Fig. 13: Venous drainage of esophagus.

3. Lymphatics from distal one-third of esophagus drain into gastric and celiac lymph nodes

The lymphatics of these three systems interconnect well. There are three types of lymph nodes according to their sites:
1. *Paraesophageal lymph nodes*: These are present on the wall of esophagus.
2. *Periesophageal lymph nodes*: These are situated on structures just adjacent to the esophagus.
3. *Lateral esophageal lymph nodes*: These lymph nodes are situated lateral to the esophagus. The lymphatics from paraesophageal and periesophageal nodes drain into the lateral esophageal lymph nodes.

> *Note*: Veins at the gastroesophageal junction are the site of esophageal varices during portal hypertension **(Figs. 13 and 14)**. Esophageal
>
> *Contd...*
>
> varices are dilated esophageal veins at the lower end of the esophagus. Esophageal varices are placed in submucosa. This is the site of anastomosis between portal and systemic venous systems.
>
> The most common cause of portal hypertension is liver cirrhosis. In cirrhosis, portal pressure increases which leads to the dilatation of veins of portocaval system anastomosis at the lower end of esophagus (esophageal varices), rectum (hemorrhoids), stomach and duodenum (gastric and duodenal varices). Esophageal varices are the main cause of serious upper gastrointestinal tract bleeding **(Fig. 15)**.

Nerve Supply of Esophagus *(Fig. 16)*

Both vagus nerves supply esophagus. Esophagus contains cholinergic receptors and vagus nerves stimulation leads to the contraction of esophagus. In LES, both cholinergic and adrenergic receptors are present, but adrenergic receptors are more, so the stimulation of vagus nerve causes relaxation of LES.

Surgical Anatomy of Esophagus, Gastroesophageal Junction, and Lower Esophageal Sphincter

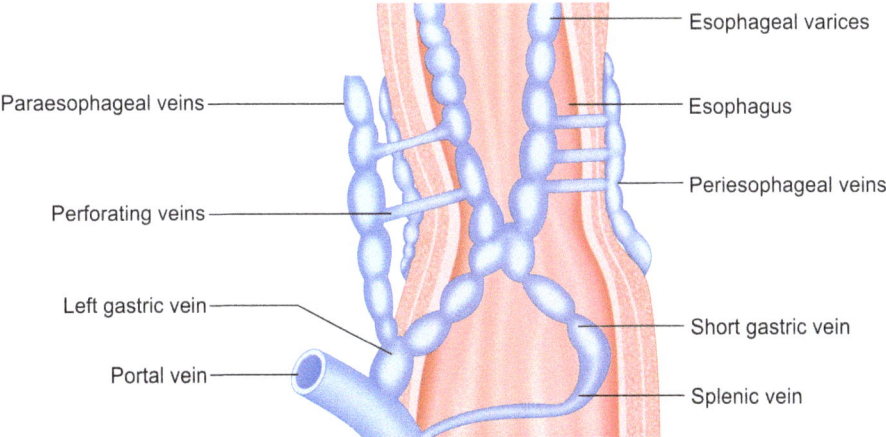

Fig. 14: Portocaval anastomosis at the lower end of esophagus, site of esophageal varices.

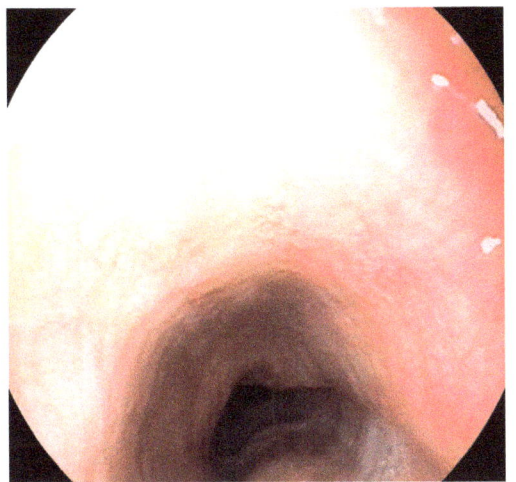

Fig. 15: Early esophageal varices.

Esophageal varices can be diagnosed by endoscopy even at early stage **(Figs. 14 and 15)**. Pain from esophagus disease may be referred to neck, arm, chest, and back. This is due to the association of afferent visceral nerve fibers from esophagus to somatic sensory fibers of intercostal and phrenic nerves.

Angle of His and GERD

The angle of His is present at the junction of esophagus and stomach **(Figs. 17A and B)**. It is an acute angle between stomach and esophagus.[9] It is between the wall of esophagus and greater curvature of stomach. It helps in preventing the back flow or reflux of gastric contents and acid from entering esophagus. It prevents GERD. It is not well developed in infants that's why acid regurgitation is common in infants. It is created by:

- Collar sling fibers
- The circular muscles around this GEJ[10]

"Angle of His" was described by a German physician and anatomist Dr Wilhelm His Jr (1864–1934). He also described the atrioventricular "Bundle of His".

Functions of Angle of His

- It prevents reflux of gastric contents and acid in esophagus from stomach and also helps in prevention of GERD.
- When air distends the fundus of stomach, then this balloon type distension pushes GEJ to the right side from the left side and closes gastroesophageal valve.

Upper esophageal sphincter is made up of skeletal muscle fibers at the upper end

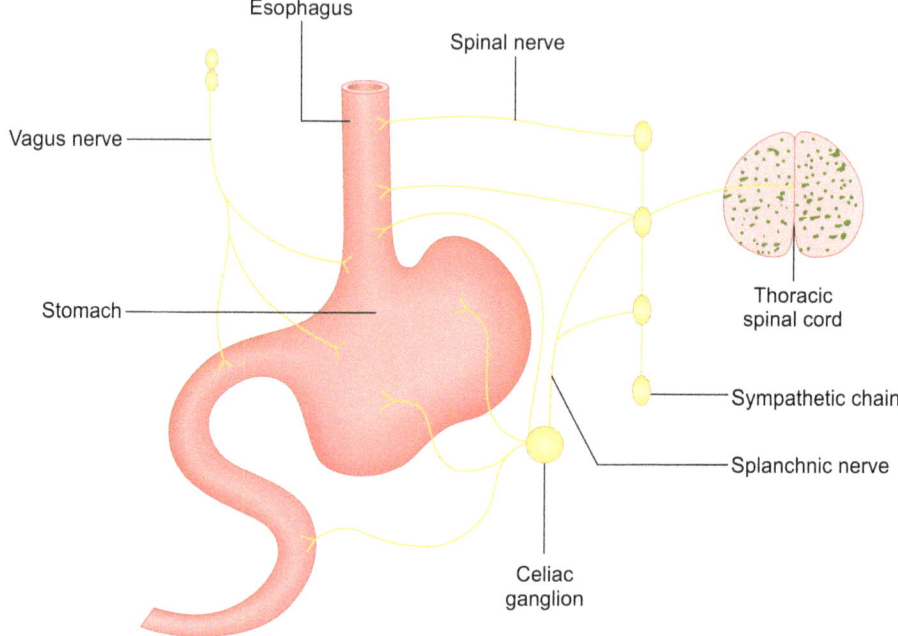

Fig. 16: Nerves supply of esophagus.

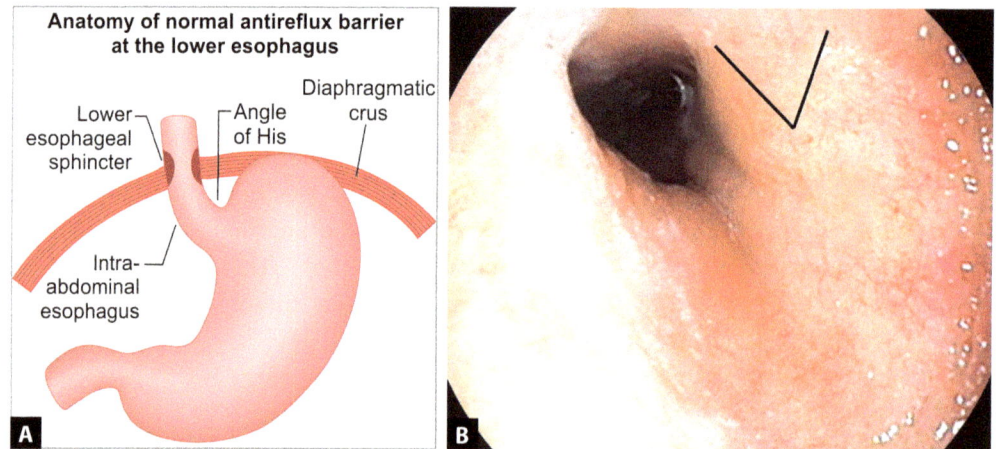

Figs. 17A and B: (A) Diagrammatic representation of angle of His; (B) Endoscopic representation of angle of His.

of esophagus. It has muscle fibers of two muscles:
1. Inferior pharyngeal constrictor muscle
2. Cricopharyngeus muscle

Note: Collar of Helvetius is the site of transition of the circular muscles of esophagus to oblique muscles of stomach at the incisura cardi (cardiac notch). It may help in preventing the reflux.

REFERENCES

1. Jacobs IJ, Ku WY, One J. Genetic and cellular mechanisms regulating anterior foregut and esophageal development. Dev Biol. 2012;369(1):54-64.
2. Serls AE, Doherty S, Par Valyar P, Wells JM, Deutsch GH. Different thresholds of fibroblast growth factors pattern the ventral foregut into liver and lung. Development. 2005;132(1):35-47.
3. Kishimoto K, Tamura M, Nishita M, Minami Y, Yamaoka A, Abe T, et al. Synchronized mesenchymal cell polarization and differentiation shape the formations of the minine trachea and esophagus. Nat Commun. 2018;9(1):2816.
4. Decker GAG, du Plessis DJ, Myburgh JA. Lee McGregor's Synopsis of Surgical Anatomy, 12th edition. India: KM Varghese Company; 1995.
5. Chaudhary SR, Bordoni B. Anatomy, thorax, esophagus. Treasure Island: Stat Pearls Publishing; 2022.
6. Fein M, Ritter MP, De Meister TR, Oberg S, Peters JH, Hagen JA, et al. Role of lower esophageal sphincter and hiatus hernia in the pathogenesis of gastroesophageal reflux disease. J Gastrointest Surg. 1999;3(4):405-10.
7. Skandalakis JE, Skandalakis PN, Skandalakis LJ. Surgical Anatomy and Technique, 2nd edition. New York: Springer-Verlag; 2002. pp. 265.
8. Skandalakis JE, Skandalakis PN, Skandalakis LJ. Surgical Anatomy and Technique. 2nd edition. New York: Springer-Verlag; 2002. pp. 266.
9. Fujiwara Y, Nakagawa K, Kusunoki M, Tanaka T, Yamamura T, Utsunomiya J. Gastroesophageal reflux after distal gastrectomy: possible significance of the angle of HIS. Am J Gastroenterol. 1998; 93(1):11-15.
10. Fischer JE, Bland KI, Callery MP, Clagett GP, Josef-Fischer DBJ. Mastery of Surgery, 5th edition, Vol 1. Philadelphia: Lippincott Williams and Wilkins; 2006.

CHAPTER 3

Physiology of Esophagus, Gastroesophageal Junction, and Lower Esophageal Sphincter

Physiology is the basis of all medical improvement and in precise proportion, as our survey of it becomes more accurate and extended, it is rendered more solid.
—John Gorrie

Esophagus is a hollow tube with muscular sphincters at both ends, from pharynx to stomach.

Esophagus has primarily two functions:
1. Transportation of food from mouth to stomach
2. Prevention of reflux or retrograde flow of gastric contents.

Esophagus transmits solid food and liquids ingested by mouth to the stomach. Cricopharyngeus and inferior constrictor muscle form upper esophageal sphincter (UES). UES is a striated (voluntary) muscle structure. UES is a high-pressure zone site. UES is approximately 1 cm in length. UES keeps the upper end of esophagus closed. It opens only when required such as at the time of swallowing or letting the gas from stomach pass out (belching). UES also prevents reflexated material entering pharynx.

Belch induces UES relaxation which is also associated with glottis closure. Stress and anxiety increase UES pressure whereas sleep decreases UES pressure.

Hydrochloric acid (HCl) is produced in our stomach to help digest food and also to kill any virus or bacteria if enter with food in stomach to avoid developing infection. The acid is mixed with gastric juice and disintegrates the food to prepare it for the digestion. The inner lining of stomach is covered with mucus which acts as a protective coat to prevent acid damaging stomach wall. Mucus helps in passage of food in esophagus **(Fig. 1)**.

■ PHYSIOLOGY OF ESOPHAGUS

Esophagus is also called food pipe or gullet. It has following functions:
- It is a long, muscular pipe which transports the food after ingestion from the pharynx to the stomach.

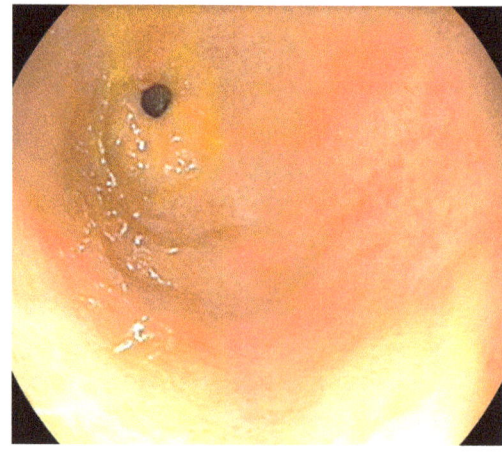

Fig. 1: Acid collected in stomach.

Physiology of Esophagus, Gastroesophageal Junction, and Lower Esophageal Sphincter

- The muscle in the wall of esophagus contracts which mixes the food well with saliva and moves it downward.
- Esophagus also contains glands which secrete mucus. Esophageal lining glands only secrete mucus and no other substance. The wall of esophagus is thin but has ability to distend and contract to allow food to enter and pass forward. The mucus thus secreted in esophagus work in two ways:
  1. It makes the passage of food in esophagus smooth.
  2. It helps avoid esophageal inner lining being damaged by reflux of acid from stomach **(Fig. 2)**.

When the food is swallowed, the UES opens and allows food to enter the esophagus. The peristalsis in esophagus moves the food down and the lower esophageal sphincter (LES) opens at this time to allow the food to enter stomach. The food bolus presses the wall of esophagus and the muscles in the wall of esophagus contract increasing local pressure but below the food bolus there is no pressure on the wall of esophagus so having the pressure somewhat low moves the food bolus down. Food bolus moves from high-pressure area in esophagus to low pressure area **(Fig. 3)**.

Esophageal Peristalsis

Normally, esophagus does not show spontaneous peristalsis. Swallowing of food and liquids and gaseous distension start peristalsis. Esophageal peristalsis is of two types:

1. *Primary esophageal peristalsis:* This type of peristalsis is started by swallowing of

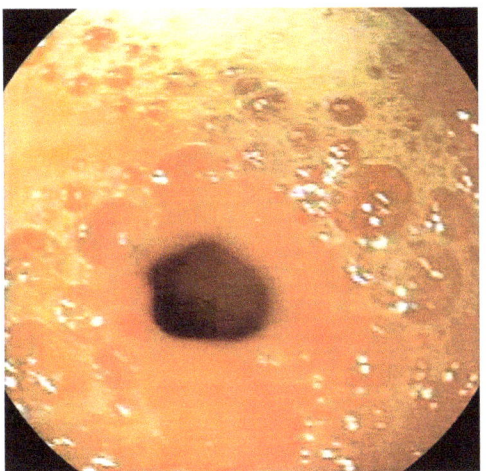

Fig. 2: Acid collected in stomach causing inflammation.

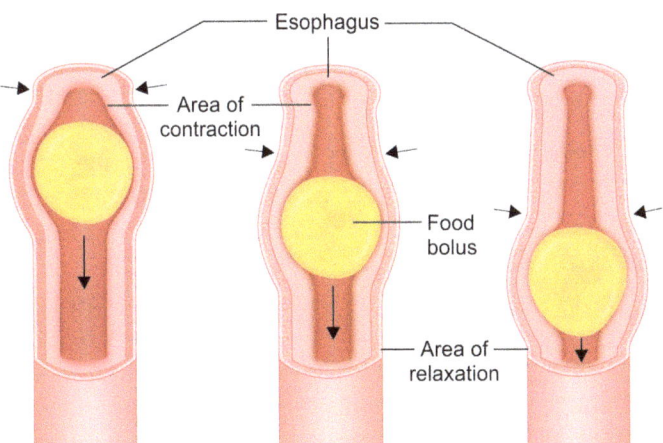

Fig. 3: Esophageal peristalsis and movement of food bolus.

food. This peristalsis involves the whole esophagus, from up to down.
2. *Secondary esophageal peristalsis:* This type of peristalsis is initiated as a response to regional dilatation of esophagus by air or fluid. It starts at the dilatation site of esophagus.

PHYSIOLOGY OF GASTROESOPHAGEAL JUNCTION

Gastroesophageal junction is actually not a simple union of the tubes but it is a valvular junction which allows the food to go down to stomach but prevents it from refluxing back to esophagus. It is actually a valve having two muscular components:
1. Smooth muscle component, i.e., LES
2. Skeletal muscle component, i.e., diaphragmatic part

This combination makes the gastroesophageal junction a competent junction. Any defect or weakness on the part of component (1) or (2) makes this junction incompetent and gastroesophageal reflux occurs. The common reason is either the tension of LES is low or it is quick, recurrent, and momentary relaxations called transient relaxation.

The gastroesophageal junction is also the site of transition of stratified squamous epithelium to columnar epithelium.

The cause of mucosal injury to the lower esophagus leading to esophagitis is due to:
- Period of contact of refluxate with esophageal mucosa
- Acidic potency of refluxate.

Higher the period of contact of refluxate with esophageal mucosa higher is the chances of mucosal injury. Similarly higher is the acidic potency of the refluxate higher is the chances of injury to the esophageal mucosa.

PHYSIOLOGY OF LES

When food enters the stomach. Churning of food happens in stomach to make it a paste so as to move forward smoothly. LES and pyloric sphincter close tightly for churning of food. If LES is not tightly closed then acid with gastric contents leaks to esophagus.

Lower esophageal sphincter is always contracted and only opens when food is passed after swallowing from esophagus to stomach. It is supplied by both excitatory and inhibitory nerves. Right diaphragmatic crus helps LES as it acts as part of it by surrounding it. When gastric distention occurs or after a big meal pressure inside the stomach increases which reduces the tone of LES and causes its relaxation. The transient LES relaxations also play a part in causing gastroesophageal reflux disease (GERD). Certain food items such as alcohol, smoking, fatty foods, and coffee also reduce pressure in LES leading to its relaxation. Muscarinic M2 and M3 receptor agonists, alpha-adrenergic agonists, gastrin, substance P, and prostaglandin F2α cause contraction. Nicotine, β-adrenergic agonists, dopamine, cholecystokinin, secretin, VIP, calcium gene-related peptide (CGRP), adenosine, prostaglandin E, and nitric oxide (NO) donors such as nitrates reduce sphincter pressure.[1]

It has been indicated by researches that only 10-mm Hg pressure is sufficient at LES to stop gastroesophageal reflux, but the resting LES pressure is approximately 30 mm Hg, as if the God knows that humans will not lead a healthy lifestyle, but will choose an unhealthy lifestyle due to their desires. So, He kept the difference of pressure threshold.

The LES is a high-pressure zone part of lower esophagus, but pressure in LES does not remain same all the time. The pressure in normal situation of rest is about 10–13 mm Hg. The pressure of LES increases

Physiology of Esophagus, Gastroesophageal Junction, and Lower Esophageal Sphincter

TABLE 1: Comparison between weak lower esophageal sphincter (LES) and strong LES.

Weak LES	Strong LES
• Overeating • Smoking • Alcohol • Overweight • Certain medicines, i.e., calcium channel blockers, sleeping pills • Fatty food • Chocolate • Peppermint • Secretin hormone • Cholinergic antagonists	• High-protein containing foods, i.e., meat, eggs and lentil, etc. • Moderate use of nuts, avocado, etc. • Medicines, i.e., bethanechol • Strengthening exercises • Meditation • Yoga

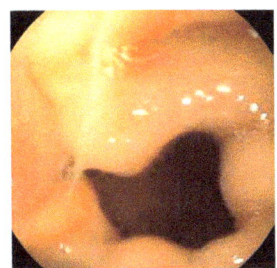
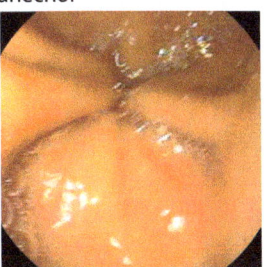

at night and becomes highest whereas it is lowest after meals. Certain factors can weaken or strengthen the LES **(Table 1)**.

Cholinergic drugs such as bethanechol have shown to increase LES pressure in normal subjects and in patients with chronic sphincter incompetence.[2]

Relaxation and opening of LES are due to the relaxation and reduction of the tone of its muscles as it does not contain dilator muscles.

Lower esophageal sphincter relaxation actually occurs due to changes at intracellular level of its cells. There is a suppression of chloride conductance and stimulation of potassium conduction. Suppression of calcium influx occurs leading to the cessation of myosin phosphorylation and muscle relaxation.[3] Acetylcholine (ACh) release leads to LES muscle contraction whereas NO leads to inhibition **(Fig. 4)**. Thus, the LES remains contracted even when entirely denervated owing to its myogenic property.[2]

Note: Neurotransmitters for LES are acetylcholine, substance P, vasoactive intestinal peptide (VIP), and NO.

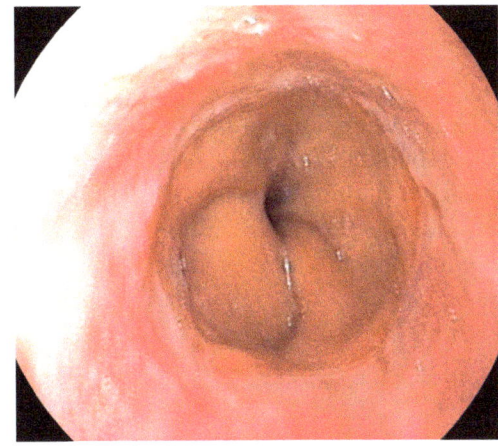

Fig. 4: Effect of ACh on LES. (ACh: acetylcholine; LES: lower esophageal sphincter)

Esophageal Acid Clearance

Esophageal acid clearance helps in reduction of esophageal mucosal damage in GERD and defective esophageal acid clearance increases the chances of esophageal mucosal injury.

The esophageal acid clearance acts by two ways:
1. Volume clearance
2. Chemical clearance

Volume Clearance

Volume clearance is the clearance of the refluxed gastric contents and acid from lower esophagus. Esophageal peristalsis is generally believed to be an important factor in the clearance of acid from the esophagus, and that impaired esophageal peristalsis is a major reason for prolongation of esophageal acid exposure in reflux disease.[4]

Motor abnormalities such as esophageal dysmotility causing impaired esophageal acid clearance, impaired the tone of the LES, transient LES relaxation, and delayed gastric emptying are included in the causation of GERD.[5] Gravity also helps in volume clearance.

Chemical Clearance

Saliva from mouth comes down and mixes with acid and mucus secreted by mucus glands of esophageal mucosa also mixes with refluxed acid from stomach. This neutralizes the acid which remains in esophagus after volume clearance. When volume clearance and chemical clearance are impaired the risk of GERD increases **(Table 2)**.

Acid clearance normally occurs in two sequential steps, first peristaltic sequences empty virtually all acid volume from the esophagus, leaving a minimal residual that sustains a low pH and then secondly the residual acid is neutralized by swallowed saliva.[6,7] ACh and NO also influence acid clearance **(Fig. 5)**.

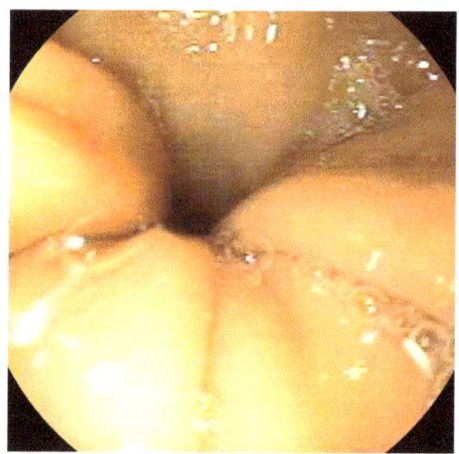

Fig. 5: Effect of NO on LES. (LES: lower esophageal sphincter; NO: nitric oxide)

A considerable body of evidence has accumulated suggesting that about half of patients with reflux disease have markedly prolonged acid clearance times. With this abnormalities of both volume clearance and salivation have been demonstrated.[8]

Nutcracker Esophagus

It is also called hypertensive peristalsis. It is a mobility disorder of esophagus. It is called "nutcracker" esophagus as there is increased pressure during peristalsis. Using conventional manometry, nutcracker esophagus was defined as a mean distal esophageal peristalsis amplitude [measured 3 cm and 8 cm above esophagogastric junction (EGJ)] >180 mm Hg in the context of normal LES relaxation.[9]

Jackhammer Esophagus

Jackhammer esophagus is an extreme pattern of the hypercontractility. Main symptom of Jackhammer esophagus is chest pain and it gets worse when you eat food. There is no known cure for this disorder. Eating semisolid soft foods help.

TABLE 2: The risk of gastroesophageal reflux disease.

Volume clearance	Chemical clearance
• Swallowing	• Saliva
• Esophageal peristalsis	• Mucus from mucus glands of esophagus
• Esophageal motility	
• Gravity	

Corkscrew Esophagus

It is a rare disorder of mobility of esophagus, there are high amplitude abnormal contractions. They are discoordinated contractions.

It is a finding of diffuse esophageal spasm in barium studies. Abnormal contractions lead to curling of esophagus like a corkscrew. It is also called rosary bead esophagus as it gives appearance of rosary beads.[10] Symptoms are chest pain and dysphagia.

Esophageal Mucosal Resistances

Esophageal mucosa is stratified squamous epithelium. It serves as a barrier between luminal contents of esophagus and deeper layers of the wall of esophagus. Esophageal mucosa repairs itself after getting damaged by acid of refluxate. Normal individuals also have GERD but not routinely with symptoms due to tissue resistance which is of three types:

1. *Pre-epithelial:* Mucus covering of esophageal mucosa is a barrier but not strong as that of stomach and duodenum. Pre-epithelial tissue resistance members include mucus covering, water layer, and bicarbonate ions. The esophagus, unlike the stomach and duodenum, has a very limited surface buffer zone, with luminal pH of 2.0 yielding a surface pH of 2.0–3.0.[11] The reasons for this are that the esophagus lacks a mucus layer and its cells do not secrete bicarbonate ions.[12,13]
2. *Epithelial:* Mucosa of the esophagus is stratified squamous. The epithelial defense consists of structural and functional components. Structural components include the cell membrane and intercellular junctional complexes of the esophageal mucosa. The esophageal mucosa is a relatively tight epithelium that resists ionic movement at the inter cellular, as well as at cellular level.

 The esophageal mucosa has buffering property as tissue resistance to cellular damage. It has both extra- and intracellular buffering. Intracellular buffering is accomplished by negatively charged phosphates and proteins, as well as bicarbonate ions.[14]

3. *Postepithelial:* Blood supply of esophagus also acts as a part of tissue resistance due to its buffering property. Under conditions of increasing luminal activity, esophageal blood flow increases, and some of the known mediators of this increase are through the release within the tissue of histamine, NO, and calcitonin gene-related peptides.[15-19]

■ REFERENCES

1. Braunwald E, Fanci AS, Kasper DL, Hauser SL, Longo DL, Jameson JL. Harrison's Principles of Internal Medicine, 15th edition. New York: McGraw-Hill Education; 2001; pp. 1642.
2. Castell DO. Physiology and pathophysiology of the lower esophageal sphincter. Ann Otol Rhinol Laryngol. 1975;84(5 PT 1):569-75.
3. Rosen RD, Winters R. Physiology, Lower esophageal sphincter. Treasure Island (FL): StatPearls Publishing; 2023.
4. Simren M, Silny J, Holloway R, Tack J, Janssens J, Sifrim D. Relevance of ineffective oesophageal motility during oesophageal acid clearance. Gut. 2003;52(6):784-90.
5. Argyrou A, Legaki E, Koutsezimpas C, Gazouli M, Papaconstantinou, Gkiokas G, et al. Risk factors for gastroesophageal reflux disease and analysis of genetic contributors. World J Clin Cases. 2018;6(8):176-82.
6. Helm JF. Esophageal acid clearance. J Clin Gastroenterol. 1986;8 (Suppl 1):5-11.
7. Helm JF, Dodds WJ, Dodds WJ, Pelc LR, Palmer DW, Hogan WJ, et al. Effect of esophageal emptying and saliva on clearance of acid from the sophagus. N Engl J Med. 1984;310(5):284-8.

8. Kahrilas PJ. Esophageal motor activity and acid clearance. Gastroentrol Clin North Am. 1990;19(3):537-50.
9. Spechler SJ, Castell DO. Clanif. Cation of oesophageal mobility abnormalities GVT. 2001;49(1):145-51.
10. Fonseea EKUN, Yamauchi FI, Tridente CF, Baroni RH. Corkscrew esophagus. Abdom Radiol (NY). 2017:42(3):985-6.
11. Quigey EMM, Turnberg LA. pH of the micro climate lining the human gastric and duodenal mucosa in vivo-studies in control subjects and in duodenal ulcer patients. Gasteroenterology. 1987;92:1876.
12. Dixon J, Strugala V, Griffin SM, Welfare MR, Dettmar PW, Allen A, et al. Esophageal mucin an adherent mucus gel barrier is absent in the normal esophagus but present in Barrett's esophagus. Am J Gastroentrol. 2001;96:2575-83.
13. Hamilton BH, Orlando RC. In VIVO alkaline secretion by ammalian esophagus. Gastroenterology. 1989;97:640-8.
14. Feldman M, Friedman LS, Brandt LJ. Sleisenger and Fordtran's Book Gastrointestinal and Liver Disease: Pathophysiology/Diagnosis/Management, 10th edition. Philadelphia, PA: Elsevier/Saunders; 2016. pp. 739.
15. Bass BL, Schweitzer EJ, Harmon JW, Kraimer J. HCl+ diffusion interferes with intrinsic reaction regulation of esophageal mucosal blood flow. Surgery. 1984;96:404-13.
16. Hallowarth ME, Smith M, Kvietys PR, Ganger DN. Esophageal blood flow in the cat. Gastroenterology. 1986;90:622-7.
17. Feldman MJ, Morris GP, Paterson WP. Role of substance P and Calcitonin gene-related peptide in acid induced augmentation of Opossum esophageal blood flow. Dig Dis Sci. 2001;46:1194-9.
18. Feldman MJ, Morris GP, Dinda PK, Paterson WG. Mast cells mediate acid-induced augmentation of opossum esophageal blood flow via histamine acid nitric oxide. Gastroenterology. 1996;110:121-8.
19. Orlando RC. (2006). Esophageal mucosal defuse mechanisms. [online] Available from: https://www.nature.com/gimo/contents/pt1/full/gimo15.html [Last accessed September, 2023].

CHAPTER 4

Histology of Esophagus

Learn to see microscopically.
—**Rudolph Virchow**

Esophagus is a cylindrical tube and consists of following layers **(Fig. 1)**:

■ MUCOSA

It is stratified squamous epithelium which is thick and nonkeratinizing and it continues upward with mucosa of oropharynx. It also contains a layer of connective tissue called lamina propria and is external to it. It contains a thin layer of muscle fibers called muscularis mucosa.

Mucosa of esophagus is pink, smooth, and even. Normal gastroesophageal junction appears as irregular line, called as Z line or ora serrata. This line separates esophageal mucosa which is of lighter color from gastric mucosa which is dark in appearance. The esophageal mucosa is nonkeratinized stratified squamous epithelium. It is a multilayer structure and has three layers which are functionally different from each other:

1. *Stratum corneum:* It functions as a permeability defender between lumen of esophagus with contents on one side and blood in blood vessels on other side, separating two entities.

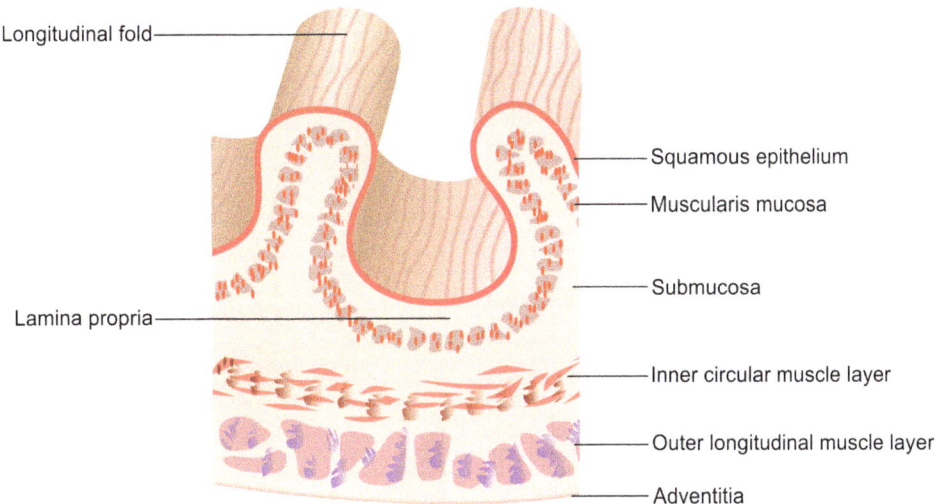

Fig. 1: Structure of esophagus, different layers.

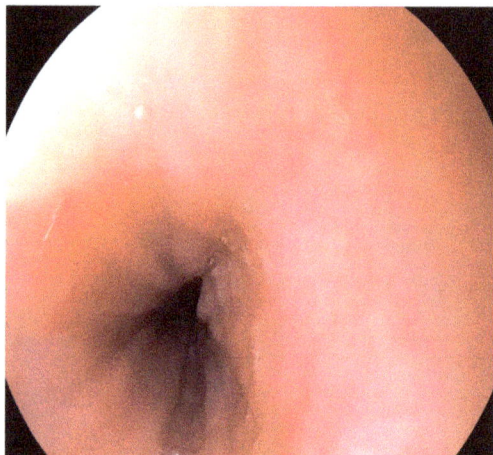

Fig. 2: Normal mucosa of esophagus.

2. *Stratum spinosum:* It has cells which are metabolically active and tissue defenders.
3. *Stratum germinativum:* These cells can reproduce.

Normal mucosa is pink and bright when inflamed becomes red **(Fig. 2)**.

■ SUBMUCOSA

It is made up of dense connective tissues. It contains blood vessels, veins, lymphatic, nerves, and mucus secreting glands. Mucosa is surrounded by a layer of loose connective tissue. The submucosa is thick and strongest part of esophagus wall structures. It is highly vascular and contains esophageal glands which also secrete mucus.

■ MUSCLE LAYER

Muscles of esophagus are arranged into two layers:
1. Internal circular layer
2. External longitudinal layer

The upper one-fourth of esophagus contains muscle layer, which is made up of striated or voluntary muscle.

In middle one-fourth, they are a combination of striated (voluntary) and smooth (involuntary) muscles.

In lower half, only smooth or involuntary muscle fibers are present.

Outermost Layer or Adventitia

It is made up of connective tissue and covers the muscle layer of esophagus.

> *Note:* The serosa is absent in esophagus and the connective tissue of mediastinum replaces it that is why the leakage or disruption of esophageal anastomosis is common due to lack of strong serosa which gives good support in suturing.

Nonerosive reflux disease (NERD) is characterized by the presence of troublesome reflux symptoms, abnormal pH monitoring, and absence of endoscopically visible lesions, but with histological changes of squamous epithelium that is microscopic esophagitis.[1]

The esophagus is having mucosal lining of stratified squamous epithelium which is non-keratinizing. The columnar epithelium lines the inside of stomach wall. The area where esophagus meets the gastric folds is called GEJ or "Z line" and normally GEJ is at squamocolumnar junction (SCJ). In GERD, SCJ moves up due to metaplasia **(Fig. 3)**.

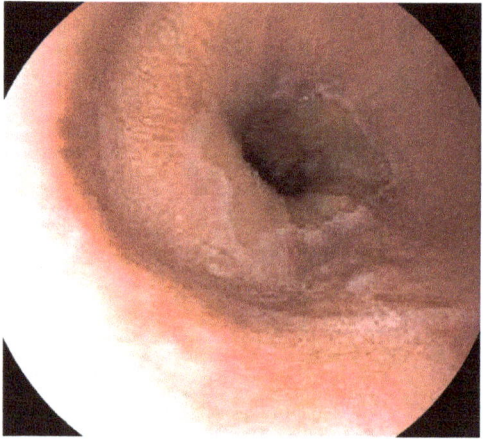

Fig. 3: Z line.

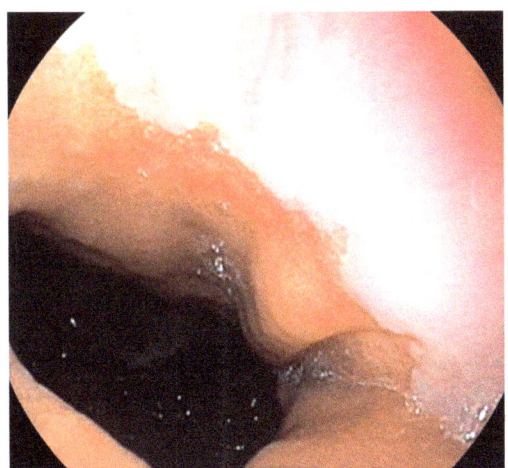

Fig. 4: Z-line distorted.

In chronic GERD, the stratified squamous epithelium gets injured due to exposure to acid and healing happens which changes squamous epithelium to columnar epithelium as squamous epithelium is not much resistant to acid attacks but columnar epithelium is more resistant to acid attack. This is nature's protective shield.

Histology of lower esophagus is important in GERD, though various researchers feel it is of not much importance. In NERD, the endoscopical picture may be normal, but after endoscopic biopsy, histology, may show mucosal injury in large percentage of cases. Histological changes in GERD mainly include proliferative changes of the squamous epithelium, such as basal cell layer hyperplasia, papillary elongation, and intercellular space dilation, but also intraepithelium inflammatory cell infiltration by eosinophils, neutrophils, and mononuclear cells.[2,3]

Inflammation due to chronic GERD causes metaplastic changes. This may lead from multilayered epithelium (MLE) to cardiac mucosa (CM), and ultimately to intestinal metaplasia and Barrett's esophagus.[4] The Z-line also gets distorted when inflammation occurs **(Fig. 4)**.

■ REFERENCES

1. Fiocea R, Mastracci L, Riddell R. Takubo K, Vieth M, Yerian L, et al. Development of consensus guidelines for the histologic recognition of microscopic esophagitis in patients with gastroesophageal reflux disease: the Esohistoproject. Hum Pathol. 2010;41:223-31.
2. Dent J. Microscopic esophageal mucosal injury in nonerosive reflux disease. Clin Gastroenterol Hepatol. 2007;5:4-16.
3. Ismail-Beigi F, Horton PF, Pope CE 2nd. Histological consequences of gastroesophageal reflux in man. Gastroenterology. 1970;58:163-74.
4. Schneider NL, Langner C. The status of histopathology in the diagnosis of gastroesophageal reflux disease: Time for reappraisal? Gastrointes Dig Syst. 2015; 5:355.

CHAPTER

5 Epidemiology of Gastroesophageal Reflux Disease

For me no good food is illuminated without acidity.
–Alexandra Guarnaschelli

Gastroesophageal reflux disease (GERD) is a common global gastrointestinal disorder. GERD is a common problem world over. No country is immune to GERD. A systematic view by ER Serag et al. estimated the incidence of GERD in US between 18.1 and 27.8%. Adults in western culture have incidence of GERD of approximately 20% **(Figs. 1 and 2)**.[1]

According to UMHS >60 million adult Americans suffered from heartburn at least once a month and over 25 million experienced heartburn daily. The pooled prevalence of GERD in the Indian population is 15.6–20.71%.[2] However, the true prevalence of the disorder could be higher because most individuals have access to over-the-counter acid reducing medication.[3,4] The prevalence of GERD is slightly higher in men compared to women.[5]

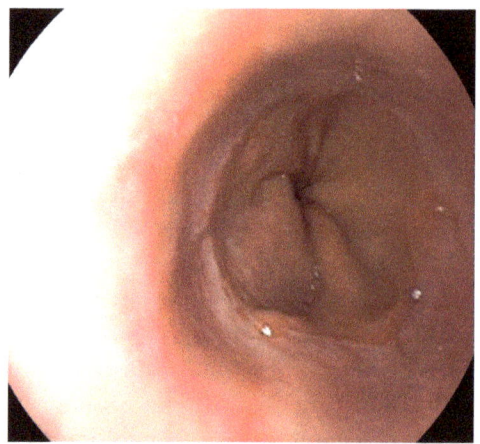

Fig. 1: Early gastroesophageal reflux disease.

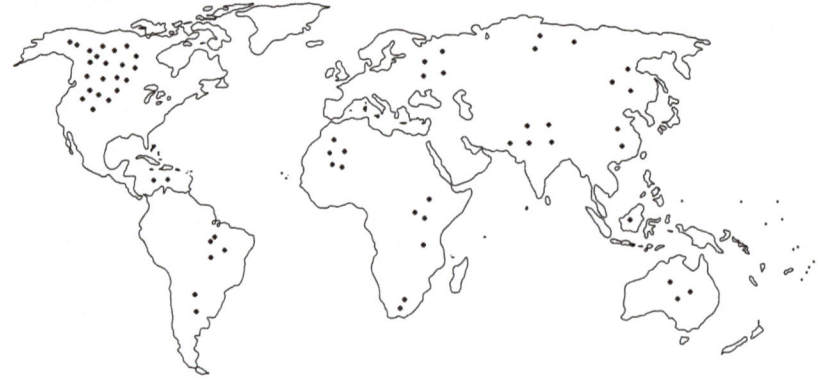

Fig. 2: Global distribution of gastroesophageal reflux disease.

EPIDEMIOLOGY OF GASTROESOPHAGEAL REFLUX DISEASE

The GERD incidence is increasing globally and it may be due to certain factors such as faulty lifestyle (alcohol consumption, smoking, and fatty foods), obesity, use of over-the-counter (OTC) analgesics and nonsteroidal anti-inflammatory drugs, sedentary habits, and stress.

The incidence of GERD is increasing world over, more in Western world. The use of antacids and proton pump inhibitors (PPIs) has become a routine and people are taking these medicines without consulting a physician. This irregular and unconsulted use of such medicines also leads to complications of GERD such as Barrett's esophagus and adenocarcinoma of esophagus. The real incidence of GERD is difficult to calculate as a large percentage of patients do not report to a clinician or a hospital and do self-medication.

It is also found by some researchers that GERD is now affecting the younger population. Takahisa et al. reported that it appears that risk factors for GERD continue to affect a growing number of adult population, but specially younger subjects, with resulting in early development of GERD.[1]

The GERD accounts for at least 9 million physician office visits in the United States each year and costs approximately $10 billion annually.[6] GERD is associated with work loss,[7] impaired health-related quality of life,[8] and esophageal adenocarcinoma.[9]

MORBIDITY AND MORTALITY BY GASTROESOPHAGEAL REFLUX DISEASE

It causes morbidity which leads to suffering, anxiety, and stress. This worsens the quality of life and mental state of the patient.

Mortality due to GERD is not usually seen, but the complications of GERD can lead to a fatal outcome. Mortality is especially prevalent in those patients who inspite of suffering from the complications of GERD continue self-medication and do not consult a specialist.

REFERENCES

1. Yamasaki T, Hemond C, Eisa M, Ganocy S, Fass R. The changing epidemiology of gastroesophageal reflux disease: are patients getting younger? J Neurogastroenterol Moti. 2018;24(4):559-69.
2. Mahadeva S, Raman MC, Ford AC, Follows M, Axon AT, Goh KL, et al. Gastroesophageal reflux is more prevalent in Western dyspeptics: a prospective comparison of British and South-East Asian patients with dyspepsia. Ailment Pharmacol Ther. 2005;21:1483-90.
3. Jarosz M, Taraszewska A. Risk factor for gastroesophageal reflux disease: the role of diet. Prz Gastroenterol. 2014;9:297-301.
4. Serag H. Time trends for gastroesophageal reflux disease: a systematic review. Gastroentrol Hepatol. 2007;5:17-26.
5. Nabi Z, Nageshwar Reddy D. Endoscopic management of gastroesophageal reflux disease: revisited. Clinic Endosc. 2016;49(5): 408-16.
6. Sandler R, Everhart J, Donowitz M, Adams E, Cronin K, Goodman C, et al. The burden of selected digestive diseases in the United States. Gastroenterology. 2002;122:1500-11.
7. Henke C, Levin T, Henning J, Potter L. Workloss costs due to peptic ulcer disease and gastroesophageal reflux disease in a health maintenance organization. Am J Gestroenterol. 2000;95:788-92.
8. Revicki D, Wood M, Maton P, Sorensen S. The impact of gastroesophageal reflux disease on health-related quality of life. Am J Med. 1988;104:252-8.
9. Lagergreen J, Bergstrom R, Lindergren A, Nyren O. Symptomatic gastroesophageal reflux as a risk factor for esophageal adenocarcinoma. N Engl J Med. 1999;340: 825-31.

CHAPTER 6

Etiology of Gastroesophageal Reflux Disease

20th century, the century of peptic ulcer illness and 21st century, the century of GERD.

Gastroesophageal reflux disease (GERD) is a common disease, caused by frequent and recurrent reflux of gastric contents with acid to the esophagus. The real cause of GERD is the incompetence at gastroesophageal junction allowing reflux to happen.

RISK FACTORS CAUSING GASTROESOPHAGEAL REFLUX DISEASE

Following factors can be considered as risk factors causing GERD:
- The most common cause of GERD is transient relaxation of lower esophageal sphincter LES (tLESR).
- High intra-abdominal pressure relaxes LES. It is a strain-induced reflux.
- Baseline low pressure at LES
- Delayed gastric emptying
- Hiatus hernia
- Drugs
- Decreased esophageal acid clearance
- *Helicobacter pylori* infection (controversial)

Age

The GERD is common in any age but it is most common in age between 20 and 30 years. GERD is also common in babies below 2 years of age. They outgrow it by 12 months of age. It does not cause any problem for babies. Persons between 70 and 80 years of age have lowest prevalence of GERD. Interestingly, several studies have demonstrated that erosive reflux disease symptoms, such as heartburn and regurgitation, decrease in severity with ageing.[1-4]

Note: GERD is increasing in prevalence all over the world and so in India. It is due to unhealthy lifestyles. Healthy, well-balanced, plant-based, and low fat regular diet is the best way for preventing GERD. Smoking, alcohol, and fatty foods worsen GERD.

Obesity and Gastroesophageal Reflux Disease

Several mechanisms have been proposed to explain the association between central obesity and GERD. Current evidence suggests that central obesity results in an increase in intragastric pressure, thus increasing the abdominal-thoracic pressure gradient, which overwhelms the reflux barrier. This leads to reflux of acidic, weekly acidic, and nonacidic material.[5]

Obesity and overweight are risk factors for GERD and therefore, body mass index (BMI) is directly related with GERD. BMI is associated with GERD symptoms in both normal weight and overweight individuals. Our findings suggest that even modest weight gain among normal weight individuals may cause or exacerbate reflux symptoms.[6]

Hiatus Hernia and Gastroesophageal Reflux Disease

In an individual with a hiatal hernia, the new position of the LES may prevent complete closure, allowing for increased backflow of digestive juices, heartburn, and esophageal damage.[7]

Smoking and Gastroesophageal Reflux Disease

Smoking is not good for your health as well as GERD. If one is suffering with GERD then one must quit it. After stopping smoking, the GERD symptoms also reduce and the risk of complications also. Heartburn is more common in smokers than nonsmokers. Smoking worsens GERD in following ways:

- Smoking increases gastric acid production.
- Smoking weakens LES.
- Smoking damages mucus lining of esophagus.
- Smoking diminishes esophageal muscle reflexes.
- Smoking reduces saliva production in mouth. Saliva acts like an antacid as it contains bicarbonate which neutralizes acid.

H. pylori Infection and Gastroesophageal Reflux Disease

The relationship of *H. pylori* infection and GERD is a controversial topic and still researchers are studying to find a connection.

Note: The role of *H. pylori* in relation to GERD symptoms and pathogenesis remains controversial.[8] The contrary epidemiological trend of an increase of GERD and a decrease of HP infection has induced the suggestion that *H. pylori* is a possible etiological factor contributing to the increase of prevalence of GERD **(Figs. 1A and B)**.[9]

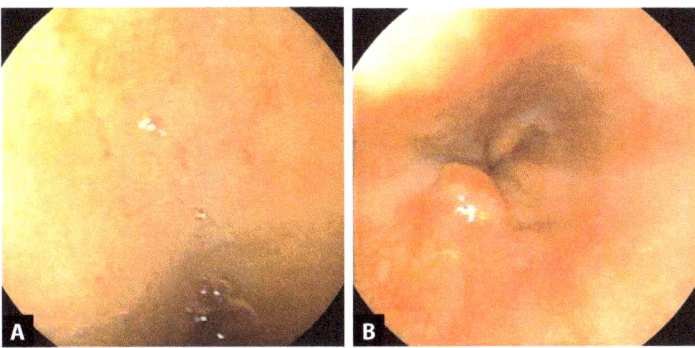

Figs. 1A and B: (A) *H. pylori* antral gastritis; (B) Erosive esophagitis in same patient.

Gastroesophageal Reflux Disease and Infants

In infants, regurgitation and spitting up is quite common and it is due to gastroesophageal reflux and does not require any treatment, but if this is associated with vomiting, irritability, discomfort, loss of appetite, and weight loss then GERD should be considered.

The GERD is common in premature infants.

The GERD in infants is not dangerous, but causes slow weight gain.

In infants, GERD or reflux usually stops by the first birthday.

FACTORS FAVORING LESRs CAUSING GERD

- Primary stomach distension (stretch receptors are more relevant than tension receptors)
- Abdominal straining
- Hiatus hernias
- Esophageal shortening
- Duration of LESRs
- Fatty diet
- Stress

Esophagogastric reflex due to a low or zero LES pressure is rare but it occurs in presence of severe esophagitis commonly.

> *Note:* In India, people chew **pan masala** very commonly. The researches have shown that further those with a habit of pan masala chewing were more likely to develop GERD compared with those abstained from the habit (Wang HY, Leena KB, Plymoth A, Hergens MP, Yin L, Shenoy KT, et al. Prevalence of gastroesophageal reflux disease and its risk factors in a community-based population in southern India. BMC Gastroenterol. 2016;16:36).

REFERENCES

1. Lee J. Anggiansach A, Angiansah R, Young A, Wong T, Fox M. Effects of age on the gastroesophageal junction, esophageal mobality, and reflux disease. Clin Gastroentrol Hepatol. 2007;5:1392-8.
2. Johnson DA, Fennerly MB. Heartburn severity underestimates erosive esophagitis serverity in elderly patients with gastroesophageal reflux disease. Gastroenterology. 2004;126:660-64.
3. Pilotto A, Franceschi M, Leandro G, Scarcelli C, D'Ambrosio LP, Seripa D, et al. Clinical features of reflux esophagitis in older people: a study of 840 consecutive patients. J Am Geriatr Soc. 2006;54:1537-42.
4. Mackawa T, Kino Sinta Y, Okuda A, Fukui H, Waki S, Hassan S, et al. Relationship between severity and symptoms of reflux esophagitis in elderly patients in Japan. J Gastroenterol Hepatol.1998;13:927-30.
5. Hazar N, Castell DO, Ghomrawi H, Rackett R, Hila A. Impedence pH confirms the relationship between GERD and BMI. Dig Dis Sci. 2012;57:1875-9.
6. Jacobson BC, Somers SC, Fuchs CS, Kelly CP, Camargo CA Jr. Association between body mass index and gastroesophageal reflux symptoms in both normal and overweight women. N Engl J Med. 2006;354(22):2340-8.
7. Hyun JJ, Bak YT. Clinical significance of hiatal hernia. Gut Liver. 2011;5(3):267-77.
8. Fatin R Polat, Sabriye Polat. The effect of *Helicobacter pylori* on gastroesophageal reflux. JSLS. 2012;16(2):260-3.
9. Vaezy MF, Swoger J. Gastroesophegeal reflux disease is in elderly. In: Granderath FA, Pointner KT (Eds). Gastroesophageal Reflux Disease. Wien: Springer; 2016. pp. 23-45.

CHAPTER 7
Pathophysiology of Gastroesophageal Reflux Disease

I cannot eat before I go on stage because I have learnt that burping on stage is not a good thing. It is all about acid reflux.
—Jessie Ware

Normally, the gastric contents do not frequently flow back to esophagus as there are barriers at the lower end of esophagus which act against reflux. These barriers are:

- *Lower esophageal sphincter (LES):* It is a collection of smooth muscles condensed as a thick cord in the form of a ring at the lower end of esophagus where it joins the stomach. It generally when empty is in the contracted state, but when the food is present in esophagus after ingestion it relaxes and allows the food to enter the stomach. It acts as a valve, not allowing gastric contents to enter the esophagus. Sometimes, especially after large meal, gastric contents regurgitate, but it happens occasionally and it is taken as a normal occurrence.
- *Crural diaphragm:* The right crus of diaphragm acts as an external LES and prevents gastroesophageal reflux.
- *Phrenoesophageal ligament:* It acts as an airtight seal around esophagus preventing reflux.

The LES and diaphragmatic crura make a good anti-reflux barrier. This site maintains a certain pressure and this pressure must be more than the abdominal pressure to avoid gastroesophageal reflux. It is observed that the gastric refluxate can cross gastroesophageal junction in either of the following ways:

- Transient LES relaxations (TLESRs)
- LES hypotension which causes relaxation of LES leading it to open a bit to allow refluxate to pass.
- Abnormalities at gastroesophageal junction such as hiatus hernia.

The TLESRs cause reduction in pressure at LES and it is for more time than when occurs during swallowing.

COMMON RISK FACTORS OF GASTROESOPHAGEAL REFLUX DISEASE

Overeating

If it is regular, causes distention of the stomach which increases the pressure on LES which gets gradually damaged and weak allowing back flow or reflux due to its incompetency.

It is observed that gastroesophageal reflux (GER) occurs frequently after a large party dinner where chocolate, caffeine, and alcohol are served with fatty large meal but it cannot be called as GER disease (GERD), it is only GER and it is only a normal physiological event.

Obesity

The same as overeating happens in an obese person.

Ageing

As we get old, our muscles gradually become less powerful and weak. Ageing is also one of the factors leading to weakness of LES, encouraging reflux.

GERD Trigger Foods

Symptoms can be triggered or precipitated or enhanced by some food items, called trigger foods, these are (**Fig. 1**):
- Smoking
- Alcohol
- Caffeine
- Carbonated drinks
- Citrus fruits
- Garlic and onion
- Spicy foods
- Peppermint
- Fatty foods

Esophageal mucosa is squamous epithelium while itself acts as barrier and protective lining to the damaging substances of esophageal contents. Recurrent and prolonged exposure of acid to this lining can damage this protective layer and cause symptoms such as heartburn and pain. So, the main reason is the period of contact between acid and refluxate with esophageal mucosa. Longer is the time of contact of these harmful substance and acid, greater are the chances of mucosal damage, i.e., inflammation, erosion, and ulceration. Therefore, the delayed emptying of esophagus and peristalsis abnormality play important role in GERD causing esophagitis, esophageal erosions, ulcers, Barrett's esophagus, and even adenocarcinoma of

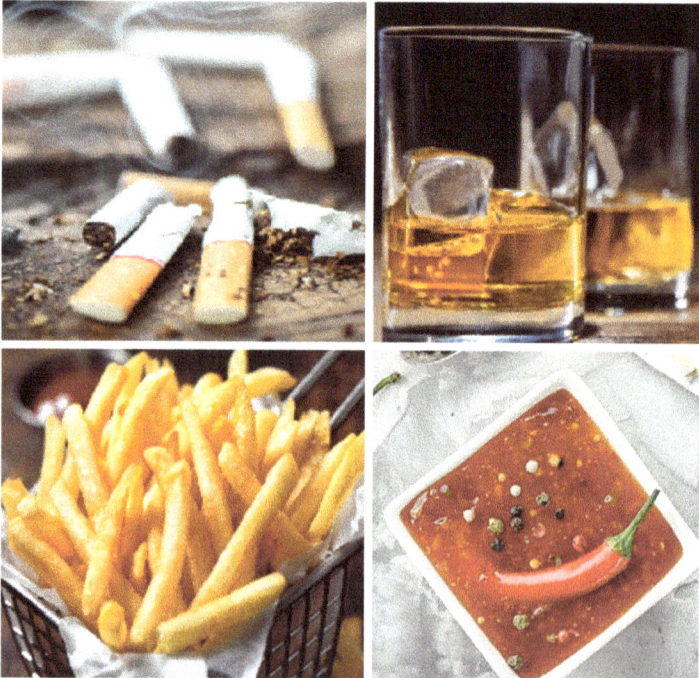

Fig. 1: Gastroesophageal reflux disease (GERD) trigger foods.

esophagus. Endoscopy and esophageal biopsy play a role in diagnosing cellular level damage.

The GERD is a frustrating illness for both the doctor and the patient as far as the cure is concerned. If GER appears recurrently and frequently then acid of the gastric refluxate can damage the esophageal mucosa and lead to GERD and its complications.

The GERD is increasing fast globally due to our defective lifestyle especially food. Nebel et al. demonstrated that 7% of those surveyed experienced heartburn daily, 14% noted heartburn weakly, and with a total of 36% having heartburn at least monthly.[1,2]

■ REFERENCES

1. Nebel OT, Fornes MF, Cast OD. Symptomatic gastroesophageal reflux: irreducible and precipitating factors. Am J Deg Dis. 1976;21:953-6.
2. Lipan MJ, Reidenberg JS, Laitman JT. Anatomy of reflux: a growing health problem affecting strictures of the head and neck. Anat Rec B New Anat. 2006;289(6):261-70.

CHAPTER 8
Clinical Features of Gastroesophageal Reflux Disease

It feels like fire in your throat.

–Sandy Pompey

Gastroesophageal reflux disease (GERD) is a common disease all over the world. GERD is so common that most of the sufferers with milder form of GERD think that it is just an indigestion and gas problem. They either use local therapy or take antacids which gives them some relief and the process of GERD goes on. If the patient starts losing weight and rapidly develops dysphagia significantly then carcinoma of esophagus cannot be ignored. This shows that GERD is a common problem, but can cause fatal disease, so it must not be ignored.

The classic symptoms of GERD were first described in 1925, when Friedenwald and Feldman commented on heartburn and its possible relationship to a hiatal hernia.[1] In 1934, gastroenterologist Asher Winkelstein described reflux and attributed the symptoms to stomach acid **(Table 1)**.[2]

The GERD produces symptoms such as esophageal and extraesophageal or nonesophageal.

COMMON SYMPTOMS OF GASTROESOPHAGEAL REFLUX DISEASE

- Heartburn
- Acid regurgitation

TABLE 1: Classical and extraesophageal symptoms of gastroesophageal reflux disease (GERD).

Classical symptoms of GERD	Extraesophageal symptoms of GERD
• Heartburn	• Noncardiac chest pain
• Acid regurgitation	• Chronic cough
• Chest pain	• Asthma
• Pain in abdomen	• Posterior laryngitis
• Belching	• Globus sensation
• Dysphagia	• Recurrent pneumonitis
• Long-standing sore throat	• Sleep disorders
• Nausea and vomiting	• Dental erosion
• Stomatitis	
• Teeth enamel erosion	

- Chest pain
- Pain in abdomen
- Repeated belching
- Pain in swallowing and dysphagia
- Long-standing sore throat
- Hoarseness of voice due to laryngitis
- Cough
- Nausea and vomiting
- Gingivitis
- Glossitis
- Stomatitis
- Teeth enamel erosion
- Bad breath (halitosis)

Heartburn

Heartburn is also called pyrosis. It is a feeling of burning sensation in upper abdomen and the retrosternal area of chest. It sometimes behaves like a heart attack. Everybody must have suffered with heartburn sometime in life. The heartburn symptom of GERD has no relation with heart, but sometimes patient may feel that he is having a heart attack and in such situation it is better to consult a clinician (**Figs. 1 and 2**).

Most of us may feel heartburn occasionally which is a normal feature, but GERD patients may feel it more frequently and even daily. Heartburn is the most common symptom of GERD. It occurs due to:

- Reflux of gastric contents with acid into the esophagus due to a relaxed or incompetent lower esophageal sphincter (LES)
- In overeating, the stomach becomes full and distended and applies pressure on LES, due to this pressure LES relaxes and opens so gastric contents with acid leaks in the esophagus (**Figs. 3A and B**).

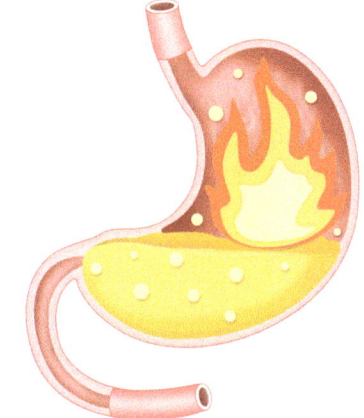

Fig. 1: Heartburn of gastroesophageal reflux disease (GERD).

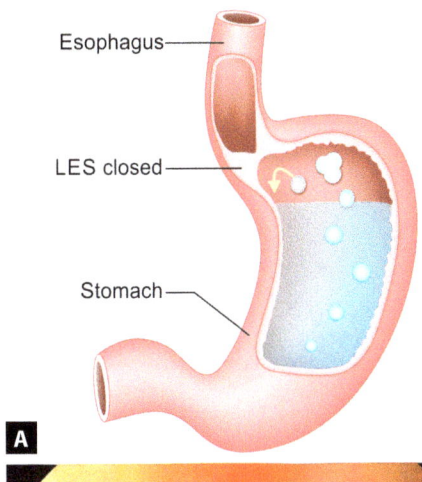

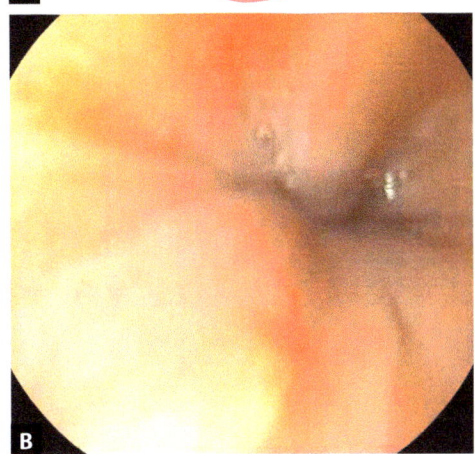

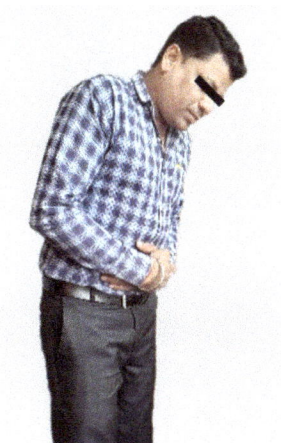

Fig. 2: Patient with heartburn of gastroesophageal reflux disease (GERD).

Figs. 3A and B: Lower esophageal sphincter (LES) is tightly closed.

- In pregnancy, the enlarging uterus with fetus puts pressure on stomach which leads to reflux.
- It is also common in smokers as nicotine relaxes LES by making it weak.
- *Lifestyle:* Heartburn is common in persons leading unhealthy lifestyle, i.e., obesity, alcohol consumption, smoking, fatty and spicy food, eating too much citrus foods, chocolates, and certain medicines **(Figs. 4A and B)**.
- *Obesity:* It also puts pressure on LES making it weak. Weight gain frequently results in development of new symptoms of GERD and worsening of symptoms in patients with preexisting GERD.[3]
- *Hobby:* Any hobby or a game or exercise such as lifting of heavy weight or bending forward which elevates the intra-abdominal pressure can lead to relaxation of LES pressure and cause reflux leading to heartburn.
- *Old age:* No age is exempted from heartburn. Although there is a tendency to reduced symptom frequency of the usual complaints of heartburn and acid regurgitation in older patients, the frequency of GERD complications such as erosive esophagitis, esophageal stricture, Barrett's esophagus, and esophageal cancer is significantly higher.[4] An elderly man may have mild heartburn, but on endoscopy may reveal Barrett's esophagus. For example, Collen et al. found an increase of esophagitis and Barrett's esophagus in patients over 60 years of age compared to those younger, 81 vs 47% **(Fig. 5)**.[5,6]

The burning feeling of heartburn starts from upper abdomen or lower chest and

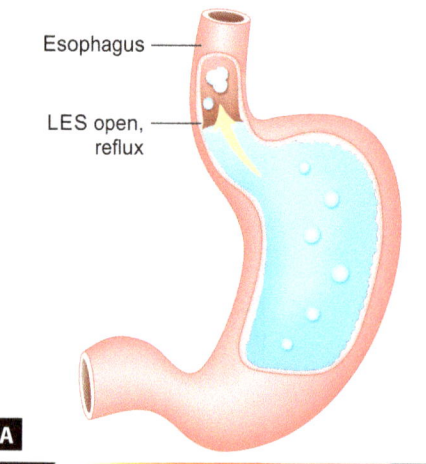

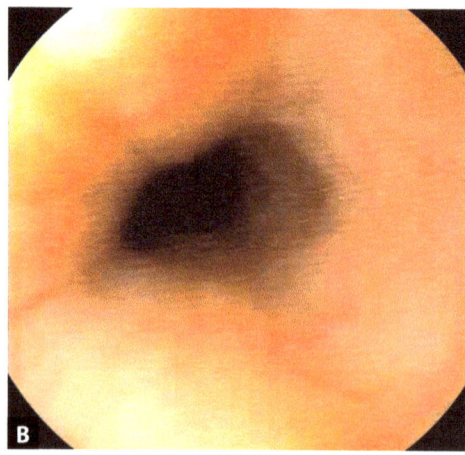

Figs. 4A and B: Lower esophageal sphincter (LES) is relaxed and open.

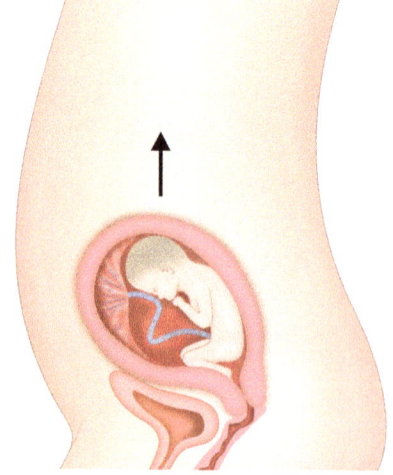

Fig. 5: Pregnant uterus putting pressure on stomach.

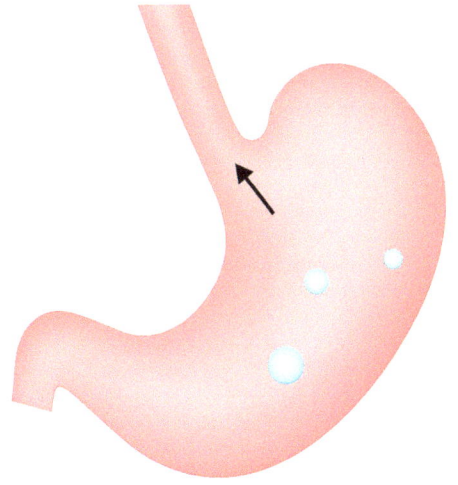

Fig. 6: Overeating putting pressure on lower esophageal sphincter (LES).

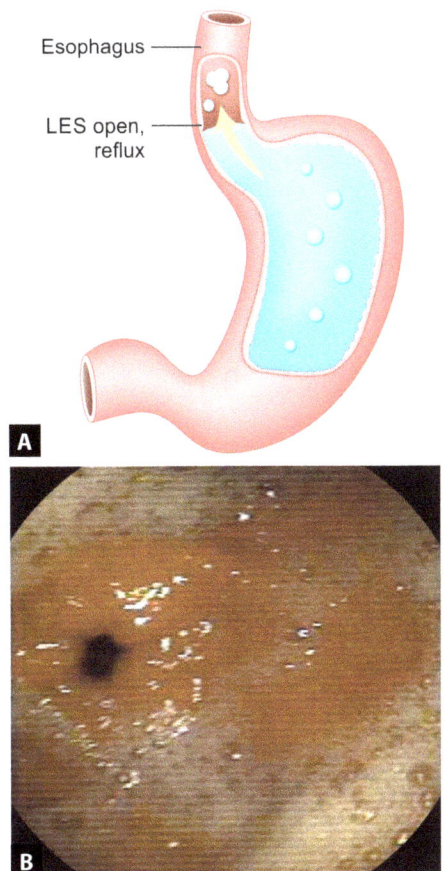

Figs. 7A and B: (A) Acid regurgitation; (B) Acid regurgitation seen by endoscopy.

moves up in chest and neck. Occasionally, it involves both arms and radiates to back. In GERD, the heartburn may be mild or severe, occasionally, or daily. Interestingly, the severity of heartburn (e.g., patients with severe heartburn may have a normal appearing esophagus on endoscopy, and those with severe esophagitis or Barrett's esophagus may at times have mild or even no symptoms).[7] Heartburn is most frequently noted within 1 hour after eating, particularly after the largest meal of the day. Sugars, chocolate, onions, carminatives, and foods high in fat may aggravate heartburn by decreasing LES pressure.[8] Overeating puts pressure on LES and weakens it **(Fig. 6)**.

Acid Regurgitation

Regurgitation of acid into mouth from stomach through esophagus gives a bitter or salty taste. It is a common symptom of GERD and commonly occurs at night. Night regurgitation of acid causes sleep disturbance. If night regurgitation becomes chronic then the chances of its complications, i.e., erosive esophagitis and Barrett's esophagus increase.

A person can spit the ingested food and rechew it or spit it out. It is called *"Rumination Syndrome"*. It usually occurs within half an hour after eating food. Exact cause of this syndrome is not known but increase in abdominal pressure can cause it. It is also considered as a psychological problem. Acid reflux or backwash occurs due to relaxation of LES and backflow of acid from stomach to esophagus **(Figs. 7A and B)**.

The most common, or cardinal, symptoms of GERD are heartburn and regurgitation. Regurgitation occurs with varying degrees of severity in approximately 80% of GERD patients.[9]

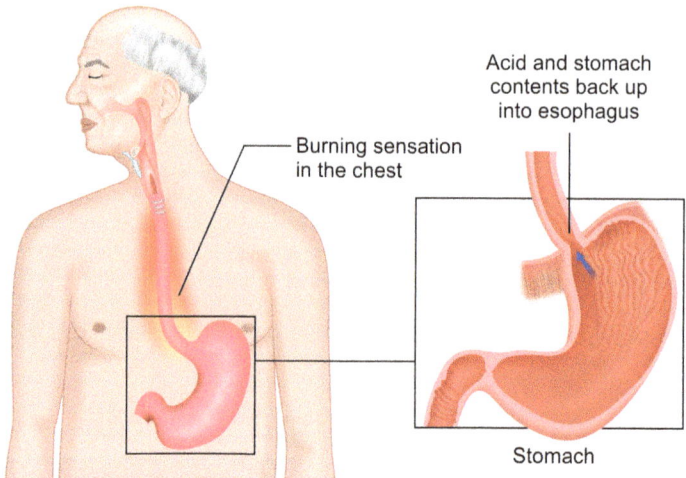

Fig. 8: Chest pain in gastroesophageal reflux disease.

Water Brash

Water brash is also a symptom of GERD which produces excessive saliva. Saliva mixes with refluxed acid causing salty taste. Person with water brash may feel heartburn also.

Reflux esophagitis develops in GERD due to acid exposure when mucosa resistance becomes low. It may lead to:
- Mild esophagitis with microscopic mucosal changes and leukocytic infiltration. No endoscopic changes.
- Erosive esophagitis—inflammation with superficial ulceration and endoscopic changes.
- Peptic stricture—when ulcers heal they heal by fibrosis and this leads to stricture formation causing dysphagia.

Chest Pain

Gastroesophageal reflux disease is the most common gastrointestinal (GI) cause of "Noncardiac chest pain (NCCP)". Following exclusion of a cardiac cause of chest pain, an evaluation of the esophagus is, therefore, appropriate.[10]

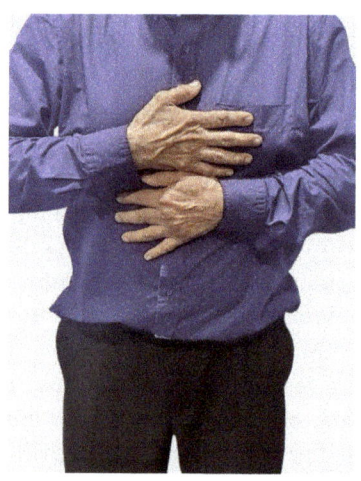

Fig. 9: Patient of gastroesophageal reflux disease with chest pain.

Chest pain of GERD may look like a heart attack pain. It is a squeezing or constricting type of pain in the sternal region of chest. It may involve the whole chest and radiate to neck, arms, and even back. The pain can last for minutes to hours. Pain usually gets reduced or disappears by antacids, H_2-receptor antagonists (H2RAs), and proton pump inhibitors (PPIs) **(Figs. 8 and 9)**.

Chest pain in GERD is probably due to spasms of the muscles of esophagus. There are chemoreceptors in the esophageal wall which are sensitive to acid. So, the exposure of these chemoreceptors to acid of GERD causes chest pain. The esophagus and heart are located at same place and have same nerve supply, therefore, there is similarity in the pain of GERD and angina pectoris. Chest pain due to GERD is the most common chest pain only second to angina pectoris.

The GERD patient can also have severe chest pain resembling myocardial infarction but this pain differs from cardiac pain:
- Usual cardiac pain is in left side of chest. GERD pain occurs in the center of chest or may occur in right side of chest.[11]
- There will be past history of classical symptoms such as heartburn in GERD case.
- GERD pain may change with position and PPIs.
- Most patients of chest pain in GERD will also be having heartburn of same type. Several studies have demonstrated that prevalence of GERD ranges 21–60% of patients with NCCP compared to patients with cardiac angina, those with NCCP are usually younger, less likely to have typical symptoms and more likely to have a normal resting electrocardiogram.[12]

Pain in Abdomen

Many patients suffer from heartburn or acid regurgitation, the classic symptoms of gastroesophageal reflux disease. Some describe belching, abdominal rumblings, or even bad breath as indigestion. Other mean pain localized to the epigastrium or a nonpainful discomfort in the upper abdomen which may be described as fullness, bloating, or an inability to finish a normal meal (early satiety).[13]

The GERD can also cause pain in upper abdomen in association with heartburn. Acid when regurgitates back to esophagus due to weakness or incompetence of LES, it irritates the lining of the wall of the lower esophagus which causes pain in upper abdomen or in epigastrium. This pain can last for hours to days **(Figs. 10A and B)**.

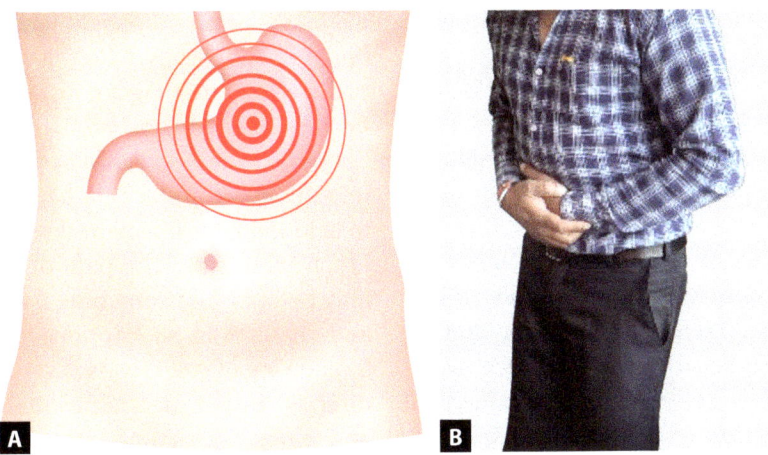

Figs. 10A and B: (A) Upper abdominal pain site in gastroesophageal reflux disease (GERD); (B) Patient of GERD with abdomen pain.

This abdomen pain may be associated with belching and bloating. It is advised that when you have abdomen pain with GERD, try to avoid fatty and spicy food, and take soft and bland diet.

Belching or Eructation

Repetitive belching is a feature of GERD. Occasional belching out of stomach gas is a normal phenomena, but if it continues repeatedly it must be investigated. Repetitive belching results from inadvertent aspiration of air into hypopharynx, which if immediately expelled, only small fraction enter the stomach. The occasional belch expels gas that is swallowed and ingested solids or liquids.[14]

Dysphagia

Dysphagia means difficulty in swallowing that may occur in the oral, pharyngeal, or esophageal phases of swallowing.[15] Nonobstructive GERD is the most common identifiable cause of esophageal dysphagia.[16,17]

Dysphagia is not an uncommon symptom of GERD. It is common in chronic cases of GERD. Causes of dysphagia are (**Fig. 11**):
- GERD induces severe inflammation in esophagus.
- *Schatzki ring:* It is a membranous ring type of structure which develops in lower esophagus at squamocolumnar junction or at Z line. It is made up of mucosa and submucosa of the wall of esophagus. A Schatzki ring does not contain any muscle. Schatzki ring is also called B ring. GERD of long standing can cause Schatzki ring and also hiatus hernia can cause it. The treatment of Schatzki ring is esophageal dilatation. It is named after the German-American physician Richard Schatzki.

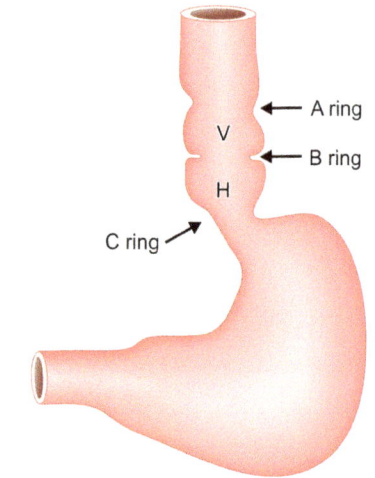

Ring A: It is above the vestibule and is transient.
Ring B: Schatzki ring
Ring C: It develops in case of hiatus hernia.
Vestibule of esophagus: It is a space in esophagus just above the stomach at the level of diaphragm and goes down in abdomen. It lies between ring A and B.
H: Hiatus hernia

Fig. 11: Rings of esophagus.

Painful Swallowing or Odynophagia

It is a problem with highly inflamed esophagus in GERD. The painful swallowing is both for solids as well as liquids. The diagnosis of odynophagia is confirmed by upper GI endoscopy. Pain can occur in throat or chest. Odynophagia may be due to viral, bacterial, fungal, or protozoan infection. The most common cause of odynophagia is inflammation of the esophageal lining due to acid reflux or infection due to bacteria or other organisms. The pain of odynophagia may be mild, but sometime it is very severe and disturbing as happens in the chest. Swallowing of solid foods is very painful and difficult. Upper gastrointestinal endoscopy and biopsy sometimes is required to rule out Barrett's esophagus and carcinoma of esophagus.

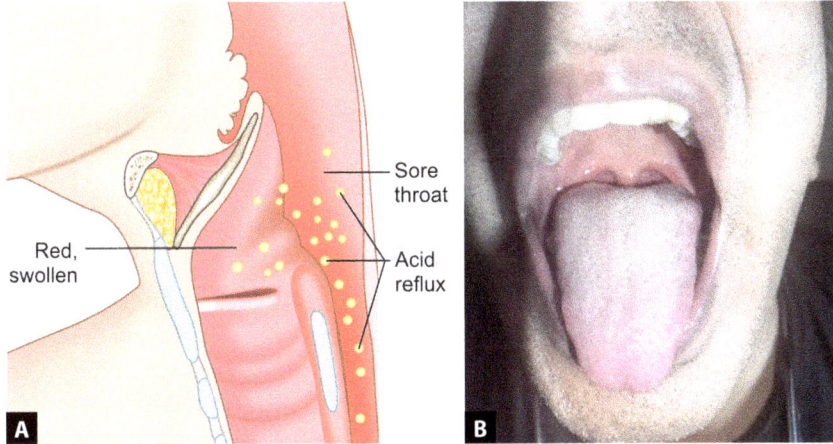

Figs. 12A and B: Sore throat due to gastroesophageal reflux disease.

Sore Throat in Gastroesophageal Reflux Disease

Acid reflux may push acid to reach throat beyond upper esophageal sphincter (UES). Sore throat in GERD gives sensation of something stuck in throat and always one tries to clear the throat. It is associated with dry cough. Acid suppressive medicines give relief in such sore throat also, but it may take 3-4 weeks to heal completely. It is advised to stop smoking completely **(Figs. 12A and B)**.

Hoarseness of Voice due to Laryngitis

The term laryngopharyngeal reflux disease (reflux laryngitis) was adopted in 2002 by the American Academy of Otolaryngology and Head and Neck Surgery and refers to clinical manifestations of gastric reflux on the upper airways.[18,19]

When acid from acid reflux crosses UES and reaches pharynx and larynx then it causes hoarseness of voice. Rest to the voice is important to treat hoarseness of voice. Hoarseness of voice may take 2-3 months or more to subside as it is due to acid effect on vocal cord which takes time to heal. To get relief from hoarseness of voice in GERD follow these measures:

- Rest to voice
- Drink plenty of water to avoid dehydration
- Use a humidifier to keep air moist.

Treat GERD with omeprazole for 8-12 weeks. In mild laryngitis the hoarseness can become alright within a week. One can take antibiotic and anti-inflammatory medicine in pain is also present.

Hiccups

It is also called hiccoughs or singultus. It is caused by contraction of diaphragm and closure of glottis. Through it is not a classical symptom of GERD, but in case of GERD, hiccups are foul.

Gastric acid suppressive medicines may give some relief in hiccups in case of GERD. Chlorpromazine and metoclopramide are used to treat hiccups.

Chronic Cough in GERD

If the reflux material from the stomach crosses UES and reaches pharynx and larynx.

It irritates these areas and causes sore throat, chronic cough, laryngitis, stomatitis, and glossitis. The mucosal damage of these areas is due to acid exposure as the mucosa of these sites is not prepared for acid exposure. The damage also depends upon:
- Amount of acid refluxed material
- Frequency of episodes
- Quantity of refluxed material per episode.

Patients who present with classic GERD symptoms and cough tends to have GERD-related cough.[20]

The GERD patients specially of chronic type commonly have cough which lingers on for weeks or even months. Coughing at nighttime and specially after dinner indicates that it is associated with GERD. It is a dry cough. One must stop smoking, avoid alcohol, caffeine, and fried foods.

The GERD patients specially chronic have throat irritation and nonproductive cough. This cough is usually after meals or at the night. These patients will also give history of classical symptoms of GERD. Approximately, 10–59% of chronic cough cases are caused by GERD.[21]

Nausea and Vomiting

Indigestion, nausea, and vomiting are common features of GERD. These symptoms usually occur after meals. Vomiting in GERD can cause sore throat and laryngitis due to the acid exposure to throat and larynx. Stopping smoking and using chewing gum may help to control nausea. If one has recurrent nausea and vomiting in GERD then must avoid fatty and spicy food and take fresh fruits and vegetables.

Try to stop smoking, try sleeping with elevated headend of bed or using 2–3 pillows to be propped up. Nausea in GERD may be mild but it may be very severe affecting day to day life.

Nausea and vomiting are present in GERD not on a regular basis, but off and on. Some GERD patients may also experience chronic nausea and vomiting.[22]

Teeth Enamel Erosion

Regurgitated acid entering the mouth in GERD can cause dental erosion. Chewing gum could induce increased swallowing frequency, thus improving the clearance rate of reflux within the erophagus.[23] The reflux of acid in GERD when crosses UES and spreads over teeth, it causes erosion of enamel. This erosion is permanent and irreversible. A patient of GERD can avoid enamel erosion by **(Fig. 13)**:
- Avoid teeth brushing just immediately after a reflux attack.
- Use sugar-free chewing gum.
- Use toothpaste which contains fluoride.

Bad Breath or Halitosis

Halitosis, or bad breath, is a complaint that often creates personal discomfort and social embarrassment. GERD has been suggested as a risk factor for halitosis.[24-27]

Bad breath is one of the most common symptom of GERD. It is due to the presence of undigested food in refluxed acid reaching to pharynx and mouth.

Drink plenty of water to refresh your breath.

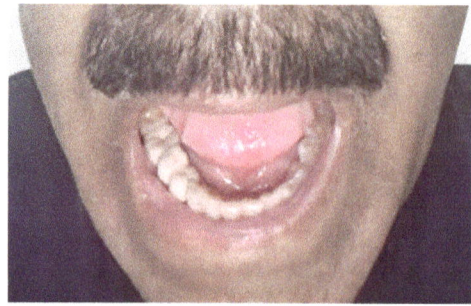

Fig. 13: Teeth enamel erosion.

Gingivitis, Glossitis, and Stomatitis

Acid reflux in GERD pushes acid in mouth and causes inflammation of gums, tongue, and oral mucosa.

> Some elderly patients suffering with GERD are devoid of any symptom or are asymptomatic. It may be due to:
> - Low perception of pain
> - Low production of gastric acid so low acid contents in refluxed material.

EXTRAESOPHAGEAL SYMPTOMS OF GERD (FIG. 14)

- Noncardiac chest pain
- Chronic cough
- Asthma

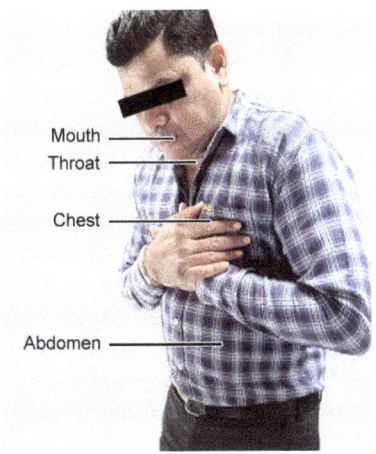

- Posterior laryngitis
- Globus sensation
- Recurrent pneumonitis
- Sleep disorders
- Dental erosion

Noncardiac Chest Pain

The GERD patient can also have severe chest pain resembling myocardial infarction but this pain differs from cardiac pain:

- Usually, cardiac pain is in the left side of the chest. GERD pain is in the center of the chest or may be in the right side of the chest.
- There will be past history of GERD classical symptoms such as heartburn and acid regurgitation.
- GERD pain may change with deep inhalation, position, and PPI treatment.
- Most patients of the chest pain in GERD will also be having heartburn at the same time. Several studies have demonstrated that the prevalence of GERD ranges 21–60% of patients with NCCP.[11]

Asthma

Asthma in GERD has strange relationship as asthma can increase the symptoms of GERD and GERD can trigger asthma. In 1966, a link was discovered between GERD and respiratory diseases, implicating GERD in the pathogenesis of asthma.[28]

Globus Sensation

Globus sensation is an overwhelming feeling of a lump or a foreign object being lodged in a person's throat. Possible causes include acid reflux or pharyngeal inflammatory conditions, anxiety, and more. A physical examination will reveal there is no object or lump present.[29]

> *Mouth:* Gingivitis, glossitis, stomatitis, teeth enamel erosion, and bad breath (halitosis)
> *Throat:* Repeated belching, pain in swallowing and dysphagia, long standing sore throat, hoarseness of voice due to laryngitis, globus sensation, and posterior laryngitis
> *Chest:* Heartburn, acid regurgitation, chest pain, noncardiac chest pain, chronic cough, asthma, and recurrent pneumonitis
> *Abdomen:* Pain in abdomen, nausea, and vomiting

Fig. 14: Extraesophageal symptoms of GERD from mouth, throat, chest and abdomen.

Recurrent Pneumonitis

The two more recognized aspiration diseases associated with GERD are aspiration pneumonitis and aspiration pneumonia. Aspiration pneumonitis occurs when a large amount of regurgitated gastric contents and acids is aspirated into the lungs, causing chemical injury.[30]

Sleep Disorders

Gastroesophageal reflux disease and sleep disturbances are both common problems. Sleep disturbances can have a significant impact on an individual's health and quality of life.[31] Taylor et al. found a higher prevalence of GI problems in those with chronic insomnia compared with those without insomnia.[32]

Symptoms of chronic GERD may be as following:

- Heartburn or pyrosis
- Acid and food regurgitations (sour eructation)
- Water brash (excessive salivation)
- Chest pain
- Coughing
- Vomiting
- Sore throat
- Hoarseness of voice
- Dysphagia
- Feeling of food caught in throat.

ROLE OF UPPER GI ENDOSCOPY

Upper GI endoscopy is used to detect esophagitis, mucosal injury, Barrett's esophagus, stricture, and carcinoma of esophagus. It should be performed for:

- When GERD is associated with alarming symptoms of complications.
- It should be performed to estimate the grades of esophagitis as per Los Angeles (LA) classification.
- When GERD patients of esophagitis complete a course of PPIs of 8 weeks of treatment.
- For taking biopsy in case of BE.

Note: Upper GI endoscopy should not be routinely performed for assessing GERD. Uncomplicated cases of GERD should be diagnosed by history of symptoms and antisecretory drug tests.

Esophageal biopsy should be taken from five sites in the esophagus. Endoscopic biopsy is not indicated when the endoscopy is normal and no abnormal signs are noted. Routine endoscopy as a screening tool is not indicated.

Sandifer Syndrome

It is a rare disorder in children, affects babies and children up to 24 months age. There is abdominal pain and unusual movements of child's head, neck, and back. Looks like seizure as baby also arches back. It is seen as a complication of GERD. It becomes difficult to diagnose Sandifer syndrome if the symptoms of GERD are absent. The paroxysmal spasms involve head, neck, and back but spare limps. It is caused by a change in DNA of the baby. Though it is a disease of young adults also rarely. It usually happens after a meal. You can prevent Sandifer syndrome by:

- Give small frequent meals
- Keep the baby upright while eating
- Burp the baby

Course of the Disease

Sandifer syndrome is a temporary condition and may go away by the time baby celebrates first birthday. When to see a pediatrician:

- When child cannot eat well
- Loss of weight
- Not gaining weight
- Symptoms worsening

THE LOS ANGELES CLASSIFICATION OF ESOPHAGITIS

It was developed by the International Working Group for the Classification of Oesophagitis, supported by the World Organization of Gastroenterology, and was first proposed in 1994.[33]

It was first presented at the Los Angeles World Congress of Gastroenterology, and hence the name of the classification.[34]

The LA classification system was published in its final form back in 1999.[35]

Grades of Los Angeles Classification of Esophagitis

Grade A: One (or more) mucosal break <5 mm that does not extend between the tops of two mucosal folds **(Figs. 15A and B)**.

Grade B: One (or more) mucosal break >5 mm long that does not extend between the tops of two mucosa folds **(Figs. 16A and B)**.

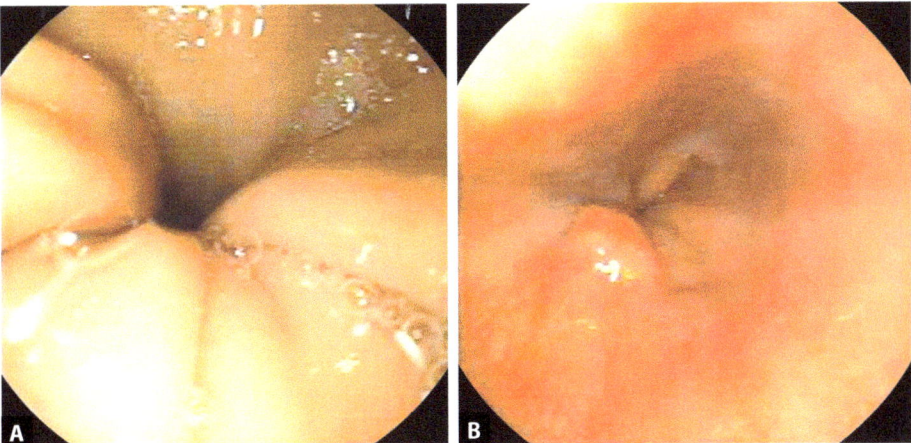

Figs. 15A and B: Grade A of Los Angeles classification of esophagitis.

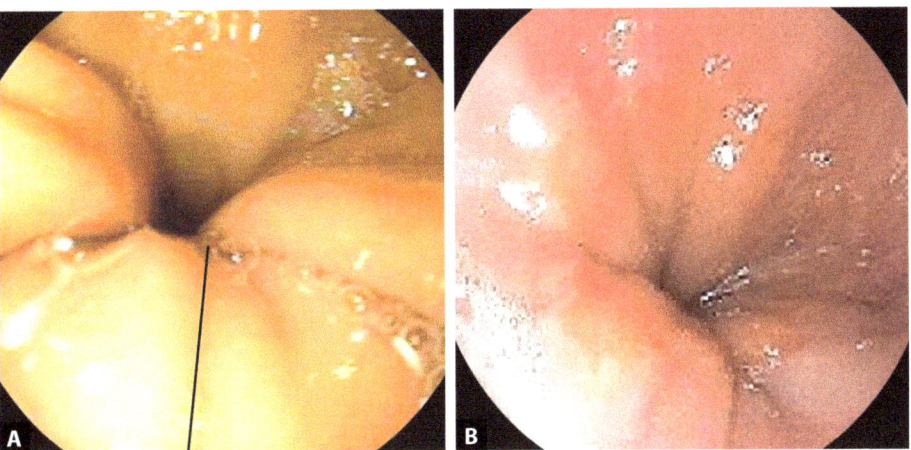

Figs. 16A and B: Grade B of Los Angeles classification of esophagitis.

Grade C: One (or more) mucosal break that is continuous between the tops of two or more mucosal folds but which involve <75% of circumference **(Figs. 17A and B)**.

Grade D: One (or more) mucosal break which involves at least 75% of the esophageal circumference **(Figs. 18A and B)**.

Advantages of Los Angeles Classification

- It is the most dependable and globally accepted classification.
- It is the most reproducible and practical classification.[36]

Classification Limitations of Los Angeles Classification

It excludes minimal mucosal changes which can be visualized by recently developed imaging methods.

Note: LA classification of esophagitis should be adopted internationally as it is validated, practical, and accurate. All endoscopist must take it as a gold standard for grading of esophagitis in GERD.

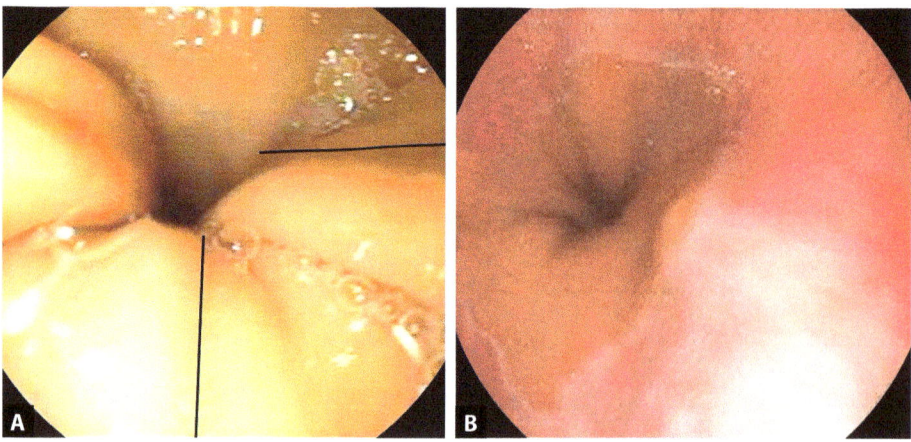

Figs. 17A and B: Grade C of Los Angeles classification of esophagitis.

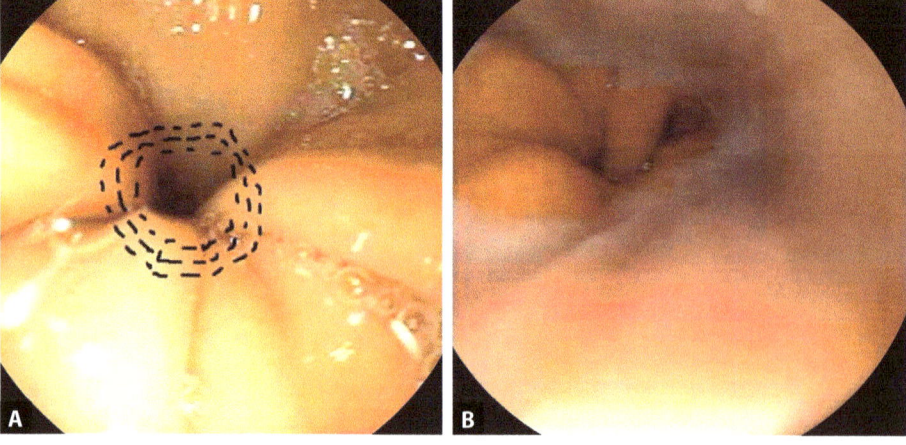

Figs. 18A and B: Grade D of Los Angeles classification of esophagitis.

> **Laryngoesophageal Reflux (LPR)**
> Gastroesophageal reflux can cause both GERD and LPR. LPR occurs when gastric refluxate with acid travel up to throat, into larynx and pharynx, LPR is also called, extraesophageal reflux or silent reflux though LPR is an acid reflux problem but you may have only laryngeal symptoms such as cough, hoarseness of voice and throat irritation, and no heartburn or regurgitation symptoms.

LARYNGOESOPHAGEAL REFLUX SYMPTOMS

- Hoarseness or voice
- Globus pharyngeus
- Chronic cough
- Chronic sore throat
- Laryngitis
- Postnasal drip

Cause of Laryngoesophageal Reflux

Relaxation or inappropriate working of both UES and LES allowing acid of reflux to reach larynx.

Factors Weakening Lower Esophageal Sphincter

- Smoking
- Alcohol
- Medication
- Foods, i.e., coffee, chocolate, peppermint, etc.
- Lying down soon after a meal
- Eating large meals
- Hiatus hernia
- Pregnancy
- Obesity

Factor Weakening Upper Esophageal Sphincter

- Normally, UES does not allow gastric refluxate to cross it and reach larynx. When UES is relaxed LPR occurs. Following factors are responsible for weakening of UES:
  - Lying down
  - Bending forward or exercising increase pressure under UES and this pressure relaxes UES allowing acid to cross it.
  - Burping causes mild to moderate weakness of both LES and UES to allow gas bubbles to pass.
  - Smoking and alcohol reduce pressure at both UES and LES and thus relax them leading the acid to reach larynx and pharynx.

It is found that LPR's responsible for >50% cases of hoarseness of voice.

Complications of Laryngoesophageal Reflux

- Throat irritation becomes chronic and affects quality of life.
- Chronic laryngitis and inflammation of vocal cords can lead to nodules formation over vocal cords and even increasing the risk of laryngeal cancer.

Diagnosis of Laryngoesophageal Reflux

- Laryngoscopy
- Upper GI endoscopy

Diagnosis of LPR is having two parts, first to diagnose LPR and then to diagnose GERD or as it is responsible for >50% cases of LPR.

TREATMENT OF LARYNGO-ESOPHAGEAL REFLUX

- Lifestyle management.
  - Stop smoking
  - Stop alcohol
  - Stop trigger foods for GERD
- *PPIs:* PPIs help in chronic acid reflux. PPIs are the most effective in LPR.

- Give rest to voice and do not shout, behave with your voice. Do not stress your larynx much.
- Surgery—fundoplication

The LPR and GERD can occur alone and also together. Treatment of LPR with PPIs may take more time to heal than in GERD. Though the relief in symptoms in LPR is early but complete healing takes a considerable time. LPR is a reversible problem. It takes 6 months or more to heal completely.

The GERD is also defined as the presence of symptoms or complications that are directly related to the retrograde flow of gastric contents into the esophagus.[37]

Actually, there is always a balance between damaging effects of refluxate and potency of protection barriers as there is always a minimum reflux, GER happening in normal individuals. This refluxed acid amount if remains below an amount causing symptoms and mucosal injury gets buffered by salivary bicarbonates remains very minimal in amount and so no symptoms arise. If defensive forces become weak or acid amount crosses safe limit, GERD happens.

REFERENCES

1. Gvanderath FA, Kamolz T, Pointer R. Gastroesophageal Reflux Disease: Principles of Disease, Diagnosis, and Treatments. Vienna: Springer Science and Business Media; 2006, pp. 161.
2. Arcangelo VP, Peterson AM. Pharmacotherapeutics for Advanced Practice: A Practical Approach. Philadelphia: Williams and Wilkins. 2006. pp. 372.
3. Rey E, Moreno-Elola-Olaso C, Artalejo FR, Locke GR 3rd, Diaz-Rubio M. Association between weight gain and symptoms of gastroesophageal reflux in the general population. Am J Gastroentrol. 2006;101:229-33.
4. Johnson DA, Fennrty MB. Heartburn severity underestimates erosive esophagus severity in elderly patients with gastroesophageal reflux disease. Gastroenterology. 2004;126:660-4.
5. Collen MJ, Abdulian JD, Chen YK. Gastroesophageal reflux disease in the elderly: more severe disease that requires aggressive therapy. AMJ Gastroenterol. 1995; 90:1053-7.
6. Chait MM. Gastroesophageal reflux disease: important consideration for the older patients. World J Gastrointest Endose. 2010;2(12):388-96.
7. Avidan B, Sonnenberg A, Schnell TG, Sontag SJ. There are no reliable symptoms for erosive esophagitis or Barrett's esophagus: endoscopic diagnosis is still essential. Aliment Pharmacol Ther. 2002;16:735-42.
8. Feldman M, Friedman LS, Brandt LJ. Sleisenger and Fordtran's book Gastrointestinal and Liver Disease: Pathophysiology/Diagnosis/Management, 10th Edition. Philadelphia, PA: Elsevier/Saunders; 2016. pp.191.
9. Kahrilas PJ. Regurgitation in patients with gastroesophageal reflux disease. Gastroenterol Hepatol (NY). 2013;9(1):27-39.
10. Richter JE. Chest pain and gastroesophageal reflux disease. J Clin Gastroenterol. 2000; 30(3):S39-41.
11. Liuzzo JP, Ambrose JA. Chest pain from gastroesophageal reflux disease in patient with coronary artery disease. Cardiol Rev. 2005;13:167-73.
12. Dumville JC, MacPherson H, Griffitt K, Miles JN, Lewin RJ. Non-cardiac chest pain: a retrospectum cohort study of patients who attended a rapid access chest pain clinic. Fam Pract. 2007;24:152-7.
13. Talley NJ, Phung N, Kalantar JS. Indigestion: When is it functional? BMJ. 2001;323(7324):1294-7.
14. Feldman M, Friedman LS, Brandt LJ. Sleisenger and Fordtran's book Gastrointestinal and Liver Disease: Pathophysiology/Diagnosis/Management, 10th Edition. Philadelphia, PA: Elsevier/Saunders;2016. pp. 247.
15. Clave P. Shaker R. Dysphagia: Current reality and scope of the problem. Nat Rev Gastroenterol Hepatol. 2015;12(5):259-70.

16. Kidambi T, Toto E, Ho N, Taft T, Hirano I. Temporal trends in the relative prevalence of dysphagia etiologies from 1999-2000. World J Gastroenterol. 2012;18(32):4335-41.
17. Cho SY, Choung RS, Saito YA, Schleck CD, Zinsmeister AR, Locke GR 3rd, et al. Prevalence and risk factors for dysphagia: a USA community study. Neurogastroenterol Motil. 2015;27(2):212-9.
18. Koufman JA, Aviv JE, Casiano RR, Shaw GY. Laryngopharyngeal reflux: position statement of the committee on speech, voice, and swallowing disorders of the American Academy of Otolaryngology-Head and Neck Surgery. Otolaryngol Head Neck Surg. 2002;127(1):32-35.
19. Wang L, Liu X, Liu YL, Zeng FF, Wu T, Yang CL, et al. Correlation of pepsin-measured laryngopharyngeal reflux disease with symptoms and signs. Otolaryngol Head Neck Surg. 2010;143(6):765-71.
20. Francis DO. Chronic cough and gastro-esophageal reflux disease. Gastroenterol Hepatol (NY). 2016;12(1):64-6.
21. Chang AB, Lasserson JJ, Kitjander TO, Connor FL, Gaffney J, Gars Ke LA. Gastro-esophageal reflux treatment for prolonged non-specific cough in children and adults. Cochrane Database Syst Rev. 2011;2011(1):CD004823.
22. Clarrett DM. Gastroespohageal Reflux Disease (GERD). Mo Med. 2018;115(3):214-8.
23. Moazzer R, Bertlett D, Anggiansah A. The effect of sugar-free gum on gastroesophageal reflux. J Dent Res. 2005;84(11):1062-5.
24. Rosenberg M, Kozlovsky A. Gelernter I, Cherniak O, Gabbay J, Baht R, et al. Self-estimation of oral malodor. J Dent Res. 1995;74:1577-82.
25. Delanghe G, Ghyselen L, Feenstra L, van Steenberghe D. Experiences of a Belgian multidisciplinary breath odour clinic. In: van Steenberghe D, Rosenberg M (Eds). Bad Breath. A Multidisciplinary Approach. Leuven: Leuven University Press;1996. pp. 199-208.
26. Bosy A. Oral malodor: Philosophical and practical aspects. J Can Dent Assoc. 1997; 63:196-201.
27. Struch F, Schwahn C, Wallaschofski H, Grabe HJ, Völzke H, Lerch MM, et al. Self-reported halitosis and gastro-esophageal reflux disease in the general population. J Gen Intern Med. 2008;23(3):260-6.
28. Overholt RH, Voorhees RJ. Esophageal reflux as a trigger in asthma. Dis Chest. 1966;49:464-6.
29. Biggers A, Fletcher J, Medical News Today. (2017). Globus sensation: Causes of a lump in the throat.[online] Available from: https://www.medicalnewstoday.com/articles/320245#what-is-globus-sensation [Last accessed September, 2023].
30. Laurance L. (2014). Consider GERD in Patients with Pulmonary Diseases. [online] Available from: https://acpinternist.org/archives/2014/03/GERD.htm [Last accessed September, 2023].
31. Roth T. Comorbid insomnia: Current directions and future challenges. Am J Manag Care. 2009;15(Suppl):S6-S13.
32. Jung H, Choung RS, Talley NJ. Gastro-esophageal reflux disease and sleep disorders: evidence for a casual link and therapeutic implications. J Neurogastroenterol Motil. 2010;16(1):22-9.
33. Armstrong D, Bennett JR, Blum AL, Dent J, De Dombal FT, Galmiche JP, et al. The endoscopic assessment of esophagitis: a progress report on observer agreement. Gastroenterology. 1996;111:85-92.
34. Sami SS, Raghunath K. The Los Angeles Classification of Gastroesophageal Reflux Disease. Video J Encyclop GI Endosc. 2013; 1(1):103-104.
35. Lundell LR, Dent J, Bennett JR, Blum AL, Armstrong D, Galmiche JP, et al. Endoscopic assessment of esophagitis: clinical and functional correlates and further validation of the Los Angeles classification. Gut. 1999; 45:172-80.
36. Dent J. Endoscopic grading of reflux esophagitis: the past, present and future. Best Pract Res Clin Gastroenterol. 2008;22:585-94.
37. Vakil N, Van Zenters SV, Kahrilas P, Dent J, Jones R; Global Consensus Group. The Montreal definition and classification of gastroesophageal reflux disease: a global evidence-based consensus. Am J Gastroenterol. 2006;101(quiz 1943):1900-20.

CHAPTER 9

Diagnosis of Gastroesophageal Reflux Disease

Diagnosis is not the end, but beginning of practice.
—Martin Fischer

The diagnosis of gastroesophageal reflux disease (GERD) is purely a clinical one. It is purely based on symptoms.

Diagnosis of GERD is extremely important due to it being a risk factor for carcinoma of esophagus. There is no test to diagnose GERD confidently, even on endoscopy 50% or more patients suffering with GERD do not show any sign. There are several other diseases which behave similarly and have similar signs and symptoms of GERD. These elements are *Helicobacter pylori* gastritis, peptic ulcer disease (PUD), and atypical GERD. The early diagnosis of GERD is also important as chronic GERD plays a role in causing Barrett's esophagus which is considered a premalignant condition.

Evaluation of clinical features with certain tests is required to reach at the diagnosis of GERD. Followings are the ways to choose from:
- History
- Physical examination
- Acid suppression tests
- Upper gastrointestinal (UGI) endoscopy
- Esophageal endoscopic biopsy
- Esophageal 24-hour pH monitoring
- Esophageal manometry

There is no single diagnostic test for GERD.

■ HISTORY

The classical symptoms of GERD are heartburn and acid regurgitation. It is rare to find in a patient of GERD without heartburn or an acid regurgitation. If heartburn and acid reflux in a suspected case of GERD absent then the diagnosis of GERD may be doubtful. GERD can usually be diagnosed based on the clinical presentation alone.[1] As many as 10% of Americans have episodes of heartburn (pyrosis) everyday, and 25% have symptoms at least once a month.[2,3] In all, GERD affects an estimated 25–35% of US population.[4] 7.6% of Indian subjects have significant GERD symptoms. 7.6% have heartburn and/or regurgitation at least once a week.[5]

■ PHYSICAL EXAMINATION

There is not much role of physical examination of the patient in diagnosis of GERD but still following examination is mandatory.
- Examine oral cavity for gingivitis, glossitis, and dental erosions.
- Examine lung and larynx for laryngitis.
- Examine abdomen for tenderness in epigastrium.
- Check for weight loss or gain, especially in pediatric patients.

TESTS TO DIAGNOSE GERD

Various tests required to diagnose GERD and esophageal damage are as following:
- pH monitoring
- Barium swallow and esophagogram
- Empirical test of acid suppression
- Esophageal manometry
- Esophageal impedance
- Endoscopic esophageal biopsy
- UGI endoscopy

pH Monitoring

A thin probe is passed to your esophagus through the nose or your mouth, the probe measures the pH level of esophagus for 24 hours. This diagnoses GERD. pH monitoring can be done wirelessly, called Bravo test.

A proton pump inhibitor (PPI) is given for 2 weeks in a suspect case of GERD and if the patient responds and then symptoms return after stoppage of the therapy then the diagnosis of GERD is confirmed. A pH monitoring for 24 hours has been considered the best modality for diagnosing GERD in patients with noncardiac chest pain (NCCP).[6]

Barium Swallow or Esophagogram

Barium swallow or esophagogram is one of the best methods to detect anatomical configuration, and helpful in the diagnosis and detailing in following conditions:
- Hiatus hernias
- Narrowing of esophagus
- Strictures of esophagus
- Schatzki's rings
- Esophageal web
- GERD with or without Valsalva maneuver

Reflux esophagitis is the most common manifestation of GERD and is the most common inflammatory condition of the esophagus. Because of its ability to provide better mucosal details, sensitivity of double contrast barium swallow has been shown to approach 90% in diagnosing reflux esophagitis.[7,8]

Though use of barium esophagography/barium swallow has decreased in day-to-day clinical practice, it still remains a valuable test for structural and functional evaluation of esophagus.[9]

Empirical Test of Acid Suppression

Empirical acid suppression tests that are performed with PPI are used to detect both the presence of acid-related gastrointestinal symptoms and GERD.[10] Some researchers feel that in NCCP which is most commonly found in GERD there is no need to do any acid suppression test but to start PPI treatment.

Noncardiac chest pain often represents a diagnostic and therapeutic challenge. Given that GERD is the most common course of NCCP, initial treatment with PPI has been proposed for all patients.

Esophageal Manometry

Esophageal manometry is the study for esophageal mobility and functioning. This study measures the contractions in esophagus and its force. Esophageal manometry is useful to assess:
- Peristaltic movements and their contraction, relaxation, velocity, durations, and force of contraction
- Pressure of LES and its contraction and relaxation.

Esophageal manometry is not done routinely for GERD which is uncomplicated.

Method: A thin tube is passed in esophagus through nose under local anaesthetic spray. The tube is attached with pressure sensors. Pressure at LES is below 10–30 mm Hg but during passage of food from esophagus to stomach it relaxes and pressure goes down below 10 mm Hg.

Lower esophageal sphincter (LES) pressure is routinely measured during esophageal manometry. However, the method of recording LES pressure, of actually taking the measurement, and its clinical usefulness remains areas of debate.[11]

■ ESOPHAGEAL IMPEDANCE

Esophageal impedance is a diagnostic test that measures the amount and type of gastroesophageal reflux in esophagus. In this test, a probe is passed in esophagus that inflates a balloon in the esophagus to measure how much pressure is required for it to expand esophagus to a certain amount. An esophagus which is stiffer or softer than normal esophagus indicates a disorder.

Upper Gastrointestinal Endoscopy

The UGI endoscopy remains the standard method to examine esophagus from inside and get details. It is good for:
- Diagnosing erosive and nonerosive, esophagitis and in its severity
- To exclude other esophageal lesions than esophagitis
- To check complications of GERD, capsule endoscopy sounds good theoretically but it's results are not much encouraging so far.

Current guidelines by the American College of Physicians suggest the major role of endoscopy is to diagnose and treat GERD complications, especially peptic strictures, and to define Barrett's esophagus **(Figs. 1 and 2)**.[12]

pH Monitoring[13]

We now have wireless pH capsules and the ability to measure all forms of reflux, both acid and nonacid. Nonetheless, ambulatory

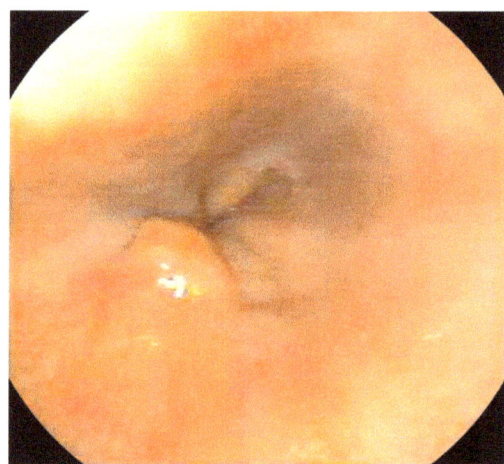

Fig. 1: Gastroesophageal reflux disease mild.

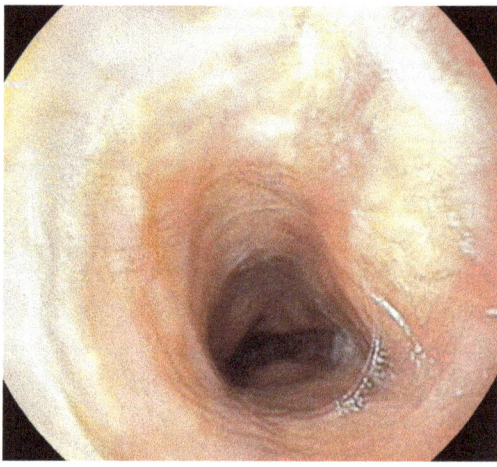

Fig. 2: Gastroesophageal reflux disease severe.

intraesophageal pH monitoring is still the standard for establishing pathological acid reflux.

Endoscopic Esophageal Biopsy

It is beneficial in cases of GERD where the esophageal mucosa appears normal and histology shows inflammation due to infiltration by neutrophils and eosinophils. Nowadays, it is done to exclude or diagnose Barrett's esophagus and adenocarcinoma of esophagus. Routine esophageal biopsy sampling in patients with refractory reflux symptoms has a low diagnostic yield. Esophageal biopsies should only obtain in patients with recurrent reflux symptoms who also present with dysphagia.[14]

> **Diagnosis of Gastroesophageal Reflux Disease**
>
> Gastroesophageal reflux disease is mainly diagnosed by history of classical symptoms.
>
> There is no role of imaging investigations in diagnosing GERD. Ultrasonography, Magnetic resonance imaging (MRI), and computed tomography (CT) are of no value for GERD diagnosis confirmation so these investigations should be avoided. Similarly, the laboratory tests are also not much useful. Upper gastrointestinal endoscopy clearly allows to see the anatomy and diagnose the pressure, severity, and complications of GERD in addition to exclusion of other diseases such as PUD.
>
> Nuclear medicine studies to study emptying time is done with Technetium–99m labeled orange juice but this procedure to study GERD has very limited role as other alternative methods are available.
>
> Barium studies are more helpful in detecting structural defects such as hiatus hernia, esophageal strictures, or neoplastic lesion than GERD.

■ REFERENCES

1. Scott M, Gelhot AR. Gastroesophageal reflux disease: diagnosis and management. Am Fam Physician.1999;59(5):1161-9.
2. Orlando RC. The pathogenses of gastroesophageal reflux disease. The relationship between epithelial defense, dysmobility, and acid exposure. Am J Gastroenterol. 1997;92:37-41.
3. Isoluri J, Luostarinen M, Isoluri E, ReiniKainen P, Viljakka M, Keyrilainen O. Natural course of gastroesophageal reflux disease: 17-22 year follow-up of 60 patients. Am J Gastroenterol. 1997;92:37-41.
4. Eisen GM, Sandler RS, Gottfried S, Gottfried M. The relationship between gastroesophageal reflux disease and its complications with Barrett's esophagus. Am J Gastroenterol. 1997;92:27-31.
5. Bhatia SJ, Reddy DN, Ghoshal UC, Jayanthi V, Abraham P, Choudhuri G, et al. Epidemiology and symptom profile of gastroesophageal reflux in the Indian population: Report of the Indian Society of Gastroenterol. 2011;30(3):118-27.
6. Fang JB, Jorkman D. A critical approach to noncardiac chest pain: pathophysiology, diagnosis, and treatment. Am J. Gastroentrol. 2001;96(4):965-8.
7. Kochler RE. Weyman PJ, Oaklay HF. Single-and double-contrast techniques in esophagitis. AJR Am J Roentology. 1980; 135:15-9.
8. Creteur V, Thoeni RF, Federle MP, Cello JP, Moss AA, Ominsky SH, et al. The role of single-and double-contrast radiography in the diagnosis of reflux esophagitis. Radiology. 1983;147:71-5.
9. Debi U, Sharma M, Singh L, Sinha A. Barium esophagogram in various esophageal disease: a pictorial essay. Indian J Radiol Imaging. 2019;29(2):141-54.
10. Vardar R, Kesen M. What is the place of empirical proton pump inhibitor testing in the diagnosis of gastroesophageal reflux disease? (Description, duration, and dosage). Turk J Gastroenterol. 2017;28(Suppl 1):512-5.
11. Marshall JB, Berger WL. End-expiratory pressure best approximates intrinsic lower esophageal sphincter pressure. Dig Dis Sci. 1990;35:267-70.
12. Shaheen NJ, Weinberg DS, Denberg TD, Chou R, Qaseem A, Shekelle P; Clinical Guidelines Committee of the American College of Physicians. Upper endoscopy for GERD: Best practice advice from the clinical guidelines committee of the American College of Physicians, Ann Intern med. 2012; 157:808-16.
13. Kahrilas PJ, Shaheen NJ, Vaezi MF. American Gastroenterological Association technical review on the management of gastroesophageal reflux disease. Gastroenterology. 2008;135:1392-413.
14. Oude Nijhuis RAB, Curves WL, van der Ende M, Herrigods TVK, Schuitenmake JM, Smout AJPM, et al. Utility of routine esophageal biopsies in patients with refractory reflux symptoms. Am J Gastroenterol. 2021;116(4): 816-20.

CHAPTER 10

Differential Diagnosis of Gastroesophageal Reflux Disease

A correct diagnosis is three-fourth the remedy.
—Mahatma Gandhi

Though the diagnosis of gastroesophageal reflux disease (GERD) is based on history taking of symptoms but sometimes the clinical features mimic other diseases than it becomes difficult to reach to correct diagnosis and here the role of differential diagnosis comes.

DIFFERENT CONDITIONS MIMICKING GASTRO-ESOPHAGEAL REFLUX DISEASE

Following conditions may have similar symptoms such as GERD and so can be confused with GERD:

- Peptic ulcer disease (PUD)
- Angina pectoris
- Nonulcer dyspepsia (NUD)
- Gallstones or cholelithiasis
- Chronic gastritis
- Hiatus hernia (Chapter 15)
- *Helicobacter pylori* gastritis
- Achalasia
- Zenker's diverticulum
- Barrett's esophagus (BE)
- Esophageal stricture
- Esophageal adenocarcinoma
- Gastroparesis
- Chronic pancreatitis

Peptic Ulcer Disease

The common acid-related diseases are GERD and PUD. Although the incidence of uncomplicated PUD has decreased in recent years in the general population, elderly population remains at high risk of PUD and its complications such as bleeding or perforation **(Figs. 1A and B)**.[1-3]

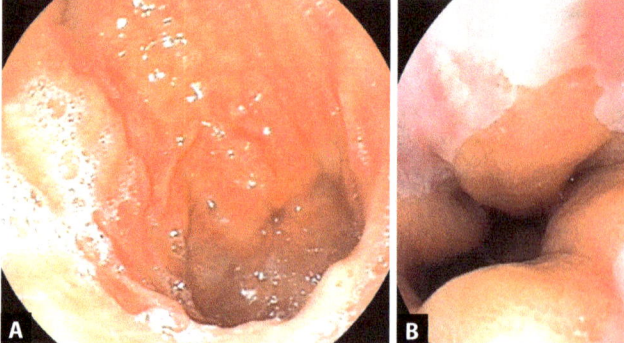

Figs. 1A and B: (A) Peptic ulcer disease, erosive gastritis; (B) Gastroesophageal reflux disease.

Gastroesophageal reflux disease though an acid-related disease but affects esophagus while as PUD is also an acid-related disease but affects stomach and duodenum. PUD is commonly caused by infection of *H. pylori* and consumption of nonsteroidal anti-inflammatory drugs for longtime and GERD is due to laxity of lower esophageal sphincter (LES) and esophageal hiatus relaxation leading to the backflow of gastric contents with acid. In GERD apart from heartburn and pain, difficulty or pain in swallowing and cough may be present which are not found in PUD. Pain in GERD is in lower parts of chest whereas in PUD pain is in the epigastrium. Upper gastrointestinal endoscopy differentiates between GERD and PUD and confirms the diagnosis.

Angina Pectoris

Chest pain is the most common symptom of heart disease and it may also be present in GERD without any heart problem.

Pain of angina is on your center of chest, it gets worse on exertion, radiates to left arm and with rest improves whereas chest pain of GERD increases on lying down or bending forward. But sometimes, according to American College of Gastroenterology (ACG) GERD, noncardiac chest pain imitates angina. Many times, patients of GERD attend emergency room of the hospital for chest pain. The heart ailment pain is usually felt as pressure on chest, tightness, and unable to breath rather pain in chest.

According to data from a large university 81–86% of patients evaluated in an emergency room for acute chest pain did not have coronary ischemia.[4,5]

Stevenson et al., says that because the heart is also located in the chest, where GERD occurs, sometimes GERD symptoms are commonly mistaken for cardiac symptoms. Similarly, sometimes cardiac pain such as a heart attack can be mistaken for GERD.

Nonulcer Dyspepsia (NUD)

Real causes of NUD are not known but following conditions are taken as risk factors for NUD (**Fig. 2**):

- PUD overlooked
- Gastritis
- Duodenitis
- *H. pylori* infection
- GERD
- GBD (Gut Brain Disorder)
- Psychological factor, i.e., stress and anxiety
- Motility
- Acid sensitivity
- Excessive amount of alcohol
- Excessive amount of caffeine

Nonulcer dyspepsia—dyspepsia, defined as chronic or recurrent upper abdominal pain or nausea, is a common occurrence.

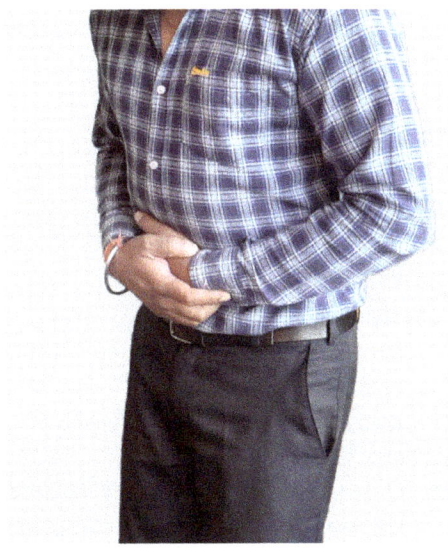

Fig. 2: A case of nonulcer dyspepsia with pain in abdomen, on upper gastrointestinal endoscopy no abnormality found.

Dyspepsia without an ulcer (NUD) is diagnosed in patients at least twice as often as peptic ulceration.[6]

The patient has a symptoms of PUD, but on endoscopy and other investigations no abnormality is detected. NUD is also called indigestion. NUD mainly affects young females, more than male individuals.

Common symptoms of NUD are:
- Pain in abdomen specially in upper abdomen
- Gaseous distension of abdomen
- Recurrent belching
- Nausea, and sometimes vomiting
- Heartburn
- Indigestion
- Feeling of early fullness of stomach while taking a meal.

Diagnosis

The NUD is diagnosed by proper history, physical examination, and following tests:
- Upper gastrointestinal endoscopy to rule out PUD
- Ultrasound of abdomen to exclude cholelithiasis.

Treatment

The NUD is treated with:
- Antacids
- Proton pump inhibitors (PPIs)
- Prokinetics
- Lifestyle changes
  - Eat small and frequent meals instead of large meal.
  - Don't lie down on bed at least 3 hours after a meal.
  - Quit smoking, no help by reducing smoking, you have to stop it completely.
  - Maintain normal weight.
  - Do regular meditation and yoga to keep stress low. Stress may be an aggravating factor in NUD. A person under stress or emotional turmoil has worst symptoms of NUD. Some physicians consider NUD as a functional disorder.
- Deep abdominal breathing or pranayama improves symptoms of NUD.
- Foods that aggravate symptoms to be avoided, such as:
  - Fried foods
  - Fatty foods
  - Spicy foods
  - Citrus fruits
- Foods that help NUD:
  - Rice
  - Apple
  - Multigrain bread
  - Yoghurt
  - Dates
  - Walnuts
  - Pears

The NUD patients may suffer for longtime in spite of the treatment.

Gallstones or Cholelithiasis

It is not clearly understood that gallstones and GERD have a link. Some researchers feel that obesity is one common factor for both the gall stones and GERD. In GERD, heartburn and acid regurgitation occur whereas in gallstones disease pain occurs in right hypochondrium which radiates to back and right shoulder.

Pain in GERD is in chest or epigastrium which may be associated with nausea and difficulty in swallowing. In gallstones, pain sometimes becomes very severe and then associated with nausea and vomiting. Symptoms occur in both conditions after meals. In GERD pain increases on lying down. Ultrasound of stomach and upper gastrointestinal endoscopy diagnose the condition correctly.

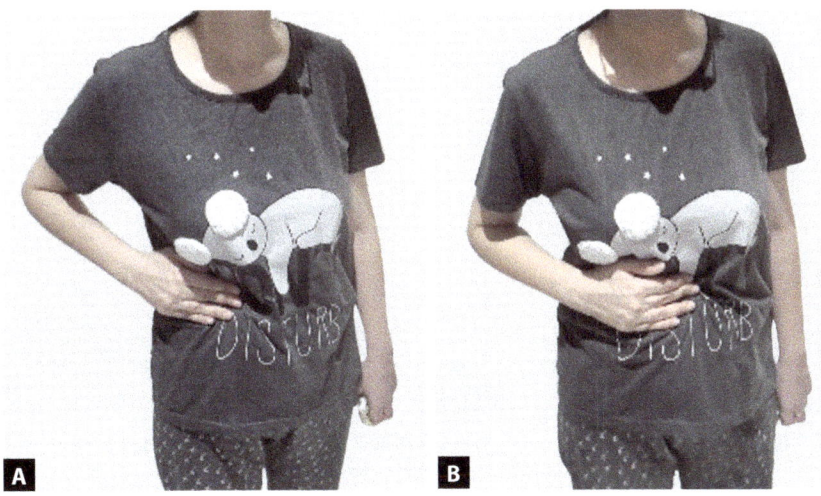

Figs. 3A and B: (A) Site of pain in abdomen in gall stones; (B) Site of pain in abdomen in gastroesophageal reflux disease.

A good clinical examination of abdomen can differentiate between pain of gall stones and pain of GERD by the pain and tenderness sites **(Figs. 3A and B)**.

Chronic Gastritis

Chronic gastritis and GERD are common gastrointestinal problems. Few symptoms such as abdominal pain, nausea, and postprandial abdominal discomfort can be present in both of these conditions. Chronic gastritis is commonly caused by infection or use of nonsteroidal anti-inflammatory drug or excessive use of alcohol whereas GERD is caused by dysfunction or relaxation of LES commonly due to overeating, pregnancy and hiatal hernia resulting as backflow of gastric contents with acid. In gastritis, there is inflammation and superficial ulcerations in mucus membrane of stomach.

Chronic gastritis patients feel abdominal pain, nausea, vomiting, and feeling of fullness after eating food even in small quantity. GERD patients on the other hand feel heartburn, chest pain, nausea, regurgitation, and/or dysphagia.

Upper gastrointestinal endoscopy is the main investigation to diagnose that the ailment is chronic gastritis or GERD.

Helicobacter pylori Gastritis

Helicobacter pylori is a spiral flagellated gram negative bacterium. *H. pylori* bacteria infect gastric mucosa causing chronic gastritis. GERD is the reflux backflow of gastric contents with acid to the esophagus causing esophagus inflammation due to exposure to acid as esophagus is not meant to be exposed to acid.

The *H. pylori* inflames various glands and cells of stomach lining, and so influencing the activity of somatostatin-producing D cells, gastrin-producing G cells, and acid-producing parietal cells. *H. pylori* gastritis causes a reduction in somatostatin. It leads to the destruction of D cells, G cells, and parietal cells of stomach lining. The destruction of D cells leads to decreased level of somatostatin which then causes hypergastrinemia which leads to hyperchlorhydria and PUD, but if continues then gastric gland destruction leads to gastric atrophy, which increases

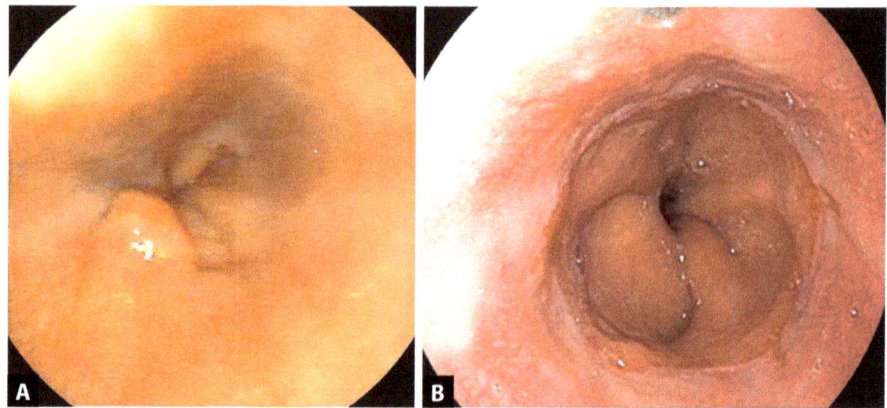

Figs. 4A and B: (A) Endoscopic view of chronic gastritis; (B) Endoscopic view of gastroesophageal reflux disease.

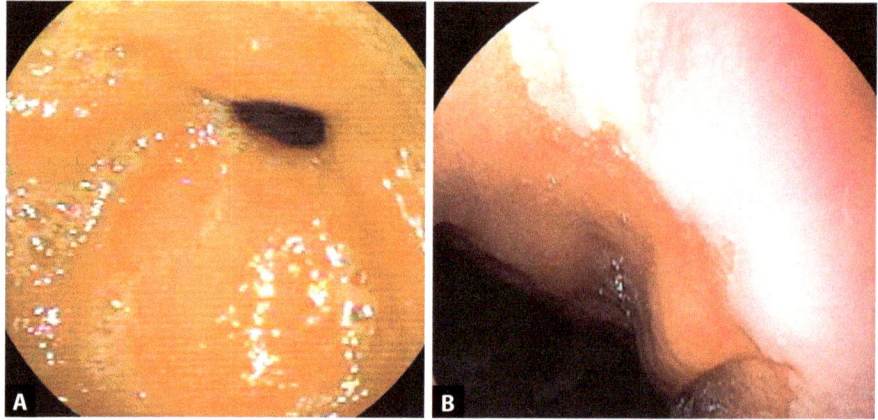

Figs. 5A and B: (A) *H. pylori* antral gastritis, rapid urease test positive; (B) Gastroesophageal reflux disease.

the risk of adenocarcinoma of stomach and this hypochlorhydria acts against peptic ulceration and also against development and complications of GERD. Chronic gastritis and GERD sometimes mimic each other and difficult to diagnose clinically **(Figs. 4A and B)**. The World Health Organization published a HRC monograph in which it stated that *H. pylori* eradication represents the best strategy to prevent gastric cancer[7] and this was recently approved for high-risk gastric cancer incidence countries such as Japan **(Figs. 5A and B)**.

Gastroesophageal reflux disease is defined as symptoms or mucosal damage produced by the abnormal reflux of gastric contents into the esophagus or beyond, into the oral cavity (including larynx) or lungs.[8,9] However a well taken history alone can prove very valuable in the diagnosis especially in the setting of heartburn and acid regurgitations which have a very high specificity (89 and 95%, respectively), and low sensitivity for GERD.[10] This can allow one to make precise diagnosis or begin empirical therapy, thereby avoiding a comprehensive and costly evaluation in every patient presenting with uncomplicated symptoms.[11]

Achalasia

Achalasia word means a condition in which the muscles of lower part of the esophagus fail to relax. Preventing food from passing into stomach. Achalasia is a rare condition where LES remains in contraction and propulsion of food from esophagus to stomach is defective leading to dysphagia. It presents with heartburn, chest pain, reflux, and dysphagia. It is a disease of adulthood. It is diagnosed by barium swallow and upper gastrointestinal endoscopy. Achalasia cardia has dysphagia for both solids as well as liquids as it is a mobility disorder whereas mechanical dysphagia patients have more chances to have dysphagia for solid only. History of sickness is more important than physical examination to diagnose achalasia. Important parts in history are:

- Is dysphagia for solids only or for both solids and liquids?
- Is the dysphagia stationary or progressive?
- Is the dysphagia intermittent or continuous?
- Is there any other symptoms associated with dysphagia such as chest pain, heartburn, regurgitation, weight loss?

The above points in history can give a clue to the treating clinician that this dysphagia is due to mechanical cause such as carcinoma of esophagus, stricture, diverticulum, or esophageal rings or it is due to mobility or neuromuscular disorders such as achalasia, hypertensive LES, or high-pressure esophagus (Nutcracker).

In GERD, there is a long history of heartburn but no loss of weight. Barium radiological study and upper gastrointestinal endoscopy are the main investigative techniques which diagnose the disease.

The LES in achalasia is hypertensive and contracted even during swallowing whereas in GERD the LES is hypotensive or relaxed.

It is observed that common symptoms of achalasia and GERD may occur in both diseases.

According to some workers, in the early stages of achalasia, chest pain or heartburn, and regurgitation commonly occur.[12-14]

Though there is a common opinion among researchers on achalasia and GERD that GERD may progress to achalasia but this is still a debatable issue as there is no sufficient scientific proof that either GERD progresses to achalasia or vice versa.

Zenker's Diverticulum

Zenker's diverticulum is also called anatomically hypopharyngeal diverticulum. It is found that Zenker's diverticulum and GERD sometimes behave similarly. Although they may coexist, Zenker's diverticulum and GERD are two different diseases, one of upper part of gastrointestinal tract (GIT) and other lower part of esophagus. It has been suggested by many workers that the association between Zenker's diverticulum and GERD is due to acid reflux to esophagus which leads to fibrosis and longitudinal shortening of esophagus causing weakness in the area between constrictor muscles and the cricopharyngeal muscle of pharynx leading to a propulsion diverticulum at this site called Zenker's diverticulum. It is common in adults and rarely in youngsters. Like GERD, Zenker's diverticulum also presents with regurgitation, difficulty in swallowing, cough, and hoarseness of voice.

Sometimes Zenker's diverticulum mimics GERD to such an extent that it becomes difficult to differentiate between the two then upper gastrointestinal endoscopy and in elder patient a biopsy is done to diagnose it correctly.

Zenker's diverticulum is named after German pathologist Friedrich Albert Von Zenker in 1877.

> *Note: Corkscrew esophagus and GERD:* Corkscrew esophagus is an esophageal motility abnormality, whose typical feature is seen in barium study of esophagus. It is a rare condition and usually occurs in elderly persons. It presents as heartburn, chest pain, and dysphagia so mimics GERD. Some workers feel that psychiatric factor also plays a role in Corkscrew esophagus. Sometimes, it becomes difficult to clinically differentiate Corkscrew esophagus from GERD.
> It is treated with antispasmodics or surgery. Operation performed for Corkscrew esophagus is multiple site esophageal myotomy.

Barrett's Esophagus and GERD

Barrett's esophagus is a complication of long-standing GERD. Every case of GERD does not develop to BE. Approximately, 10% of people suffering from GERD develop BE, but the incidence differs from country to country. The importance of BE is that it can lead to the development of adenocarcinoma of esophagus which has poor prognosis and unfortunately the incidence of adenocarcinoma has increased globally.

It is difficult to diagnose BE correctly by only history from a patient of GERD. It is also not clear that how long it takes GERD to progress to BE but studies show that at last >10 years are required to develop BE in patients of GERD. Periodic upper gastrointestinal endoscopy is required with biopsy and if changes are not there, it can be repeated at 3–5 years interval. There are no specific symptoms of BE. The symptoms such as heartburn, chest pain, regurgitation, and cough are common symptoms of both GERD and BE. It is not easy to diagnose that BE has developed in a patient with chronic GERD. Upper gastrointestinal endoscopy with biopsy is the gold standard to confirm BE. Whereas, 24-hour pH manometry is standard method to identify GERD.

Esophageal Stricture

Esophageal stricture is the abnormal narrowing of the lumen of esophagus. It can be caused by various factors. Esophageal strictures can be caused by:
- Cancer of esophagus
- GERD
- Eosinophilic esophagitis
- Accidental swallowing of chemicals
- Radiation therapy
- Operation on esophagus

Symptoms of esophageal strictures are:
- Dysphagia
- Burning sensation or pain in neck
- Feeling of sticking of food in esophagus
- Choking
- Regurgitation
- Weight loss

Esophageal strictures are diagnosed by barium study and upper gastrointestinal endoscopy. Long-standing cases of GERD may cause esophageal strictures as the damaged mucosa of lower esophagus heals with scarring that leads to strictures.

In esophageal stricture, the dysphagia is a prominent symptoms whereas in GERD heartburn is the main symptom. Regurgitation with vomiting is more common in esophageal strictures.

Esophageal Adenocarcinoma

In GERD, heartburn and chest pain are present but in case of adenocarcinoma of esophagus, dysphagia and weight loss are present. Even in long-standing cases of GERD, weight loss is not seen.

Upper gastrointestinal endoscopy is the main investigation to differentiate between two illness and confirm the diagnosis.

Dysphagia, pain in center of chest, and loss of weight are important features of adenocarcinomal of esophagus. GERD can turn to BE after suffering for long and BE is a precancerous condition which converts to adenocarcinoma of esophagus. BE is the most common precancerous condition of esophagus. So, GERD is a risk factor for adenocarcinoma of esophagus, so if a patient of GERD complains of long-standing increased severity of chest pain, recurrent vomiting, significant weakness, and weight loss, the individual must be put up for upper gastrointestinal endoscopy and the biopsy will prove cancer even if early and not observed on endoscopy.

The most common site of esophageal cancer is lower esophagus so the clinical picture mimics GERD. It has been observed that obesity is a risk factor for GERD as it presses stomach and acid with stomach contents is pushed up in esophagus which may lead to precancerous condition and then adenocarcinoma of esophagus. So, keeping weight within normal ranges is a way to prevent adenocarcinoma of esophagus.

Upper gastrointestinal endoscopy and biopsy in GERD show no dysplasia then once in 3–5 years endoscopy should be done but if dysplasia presents then endoscopy should be done yearly.

Gastroparesis

Gastroparesis is a condition where the stomach empties the contents slowly. This delayed emptying of stomach is due to muscle weakness and is probably due to damage to the nerves controlling the muscles of stomach or the paralysis of stomach. It is a functional disorder. Gastroparesis can affect digestion. It presents nausea, vomiting, and abdominal pain.

Gastroparesis can be defined as paralysis of stomach, leading to a delayed rate of emptying of a standard test meal. Approximately, about 90% of the patients with gastroparesis have either diabetic, postsurgical or idiopathic gastroparesis, but the less common forms of obstructive and ischemic gastroparesis are important because they are reversible.[15]

The GERD patients have heartburn commonly which is not so prominent in gastroparesis and GERD patients have pain in upper abdomen and gastroparesis patients have abdominal pain but a bit lower site.

The GERD patients also have delayed gastric emptying but not all patients but in gastroparesis most of the patients have delayed gastric emptying due to paralysis of the stomach. Some patients of GERD also complain of postprandial fullness and mimic gastroparesis. GERD is treated with PPIs and they are quite effective in controlling the symptoms but in gastroparesis PPIs have no role.

Chronic Pancreatitis

The GERD and chronic pancreatitis are the diseases of GIT but of two different organs. GERD symptoms are due to backflow of acid and gastric contents to esophagus causing heartburn, pain in upper abdomen or chest also, regurgitation and difficulty and pain in swallowing food. Chronic pancreatitis is the chronic inflammation of pancreas leading to abdominal pain, nausea, vomiting, and fever. The pain in pancreatitis is usually very severe.

Both the GERD and chronic pancreatitis must be treated well and must not be ignored and if untreated both the GERD and pancreatitis can become serious.

REFERENCES

1. Malfertheiner P, Chan FK, McColl KE. Peptic ulcer disease. Lancet. 2009;37(9699):1949-61.
2. Pilotto A. Helicobacter pylori associated peptic ulcer disease in older patients. Current management strategies. Drugs Aging. 2001;18(7):487-94.
3. Lau JY, Sung J, Hill C, Hinderson C, Howden CW, Metz DC. Systematic review of the epidemiology of complicated peptic ulcer disease: incidence, recurrence, risk factors and mortality. Digestion. 2011; 84(2):102-113.
4. Udelson JE, Beshanksy JR, Handler J, Heller GV, Handell C, Pope JH, et al. Myocardial perfusion imaging for evolution and triage of patients with suspected acute cardiac ischemia: a randomized controlled trial. JAMA. 2002;288:2693-700.
5. Katz PO, Castel DO. Approach to the patient with unexplained chest pain. Am J Gastroenterol. 2000;95:54-8.
6. Talley NJ, Phillips SF. Nonulcer dyspepsia: Potential causes and pathophysiology. Ann Intern Med. 1988;108(6):865-79.
7. IARC Helicobacter Working Group. Helicobacter pylori eradication as a strategy for preventing gastric cancer—IARC Working Group Reports Vol 8. Lyon, France: WHO Press; 2014.
8. De Valult KR, Castell DO. Updated guidelines for the diagnosis and management of gastroesophageal reflux disease. Am J Gastroenterol. 2013;108:308-28.
9. Dent J, El-Serag HB, Wallander MA, Johansson S. Epidemiology of gastroesophageal reflux disease: a systematic review. Gut. 2005; 54:710-7.
10. Klauser AG, Schindlbeck ME, Muller-Lissner SA. Symptom in gastroesophageal reflux disease. Lancet. 1990;335:205-8.
11. Giannini EG, Zentilin P, Dulbecco P, Vigneri S, Scarlata P, Savrino V. Management strategy for patients with gastroesophageal reflux disease: A comparison between empirical treatment with esomeprazole and endoscopy oriented treatment. Am J Gastroenterol. 2008:103:267-75.
12. Olsen AM, Holman CB, Anderson HA. The diagnosis of cardiospasm. Dis Chest. 1953;23:477-98.
13. Adams CW, Brain RH, Ellis FG, Kauntze R, Trounce JR. Achalasia of the cardiac Guys. Hosp Resp. 1961;110:191-236.
14. Goldenberg SP, Burrell M, Fette GG, Vos C, Tranbe M. Classic and vigorous achalasia: a comparison of manometric, radiographic, and clinical findings. Gastroenterology. 1991;101:743-8.
15. Feldman M, Friedman LS, Brandt LJ. Sleisenger and Fordtran's book "Gastro-intestinal and Liver Disease", 10th edition, Philadelphia: Saunders Elsevier; 2016. pp. 829.

CHAPTER 11

Complications of Gastroesophageal Reflux Disease

Life doesn't have complications if you do not complicate it.
—Fadhili G. Mwike

Gastroesophageal reflux disease (GERD) complications are commonly present in elderly patients. Quality of life and well-being are severely affected in most of the patients with chronic GERD.

Left untreated GERD can result in several serious complications, including esophagitis and Barrett's esophagus. Esophagitis can vary widely in severity with severe cases resulting in extensive erosions, ulcerations, and narrowing of the esophagus.[1] Esophagitis may also lead to gastrointestinal (GI) bleeding.[2]

COMPLICATIONS OF GASTROESOPHAGEAL REFLUX DISEASE

Following are the complications of GERD:
- Esophagitis
- Barrett's esophagus (Chapter 14)
- Esophageal strictures (Chapter 10)
- Esophageal carcinoma
- Hemorrhage
- Ulcers
- Perforation

Esophagitis

Esophagitis is the inflammation of esophagus causing heartburn, chest pain, and painful swallowing. The common symptoms of esophagitis are:
- Painful swallowing
- Dysphagia
- Feeling of food impaction in chest
- Heartburn
- Chest pain

Esophagitis is most commonly caused by acid reflux, but there are other causes also:
- Reflux esophagitis
- Eosinophilic esophagitis (EOE)
- Lymphocytic esophagitis
- Infectious esophagitis
- Drug-induced esophagitis

Reflux Esophagitis

When gastroesophageal junction becomes incompetent, reflux of gastric contents to the esophagus occurs, which if recurrent and frequent leads to damage of the mucosal lining of the lower esophagus leading to esophagitis.

Eosinophilic Esophagitis (EOE)

The esophagus is normally devoid of eosinophils, so the finding of esophageal eosinophils denotes pathology. The etiology of eosinophils esophagitis is poorly

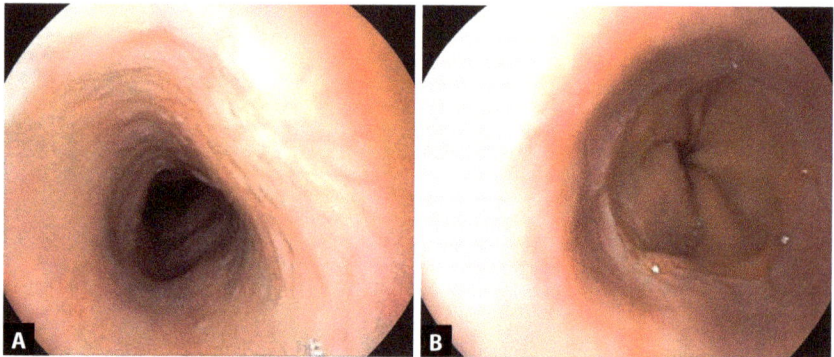

Figs. 1A and B: (A) Mild esophagitis due to gastroesophageal reflux disease (GERD); (B) Severe esophagitis due to GERD.

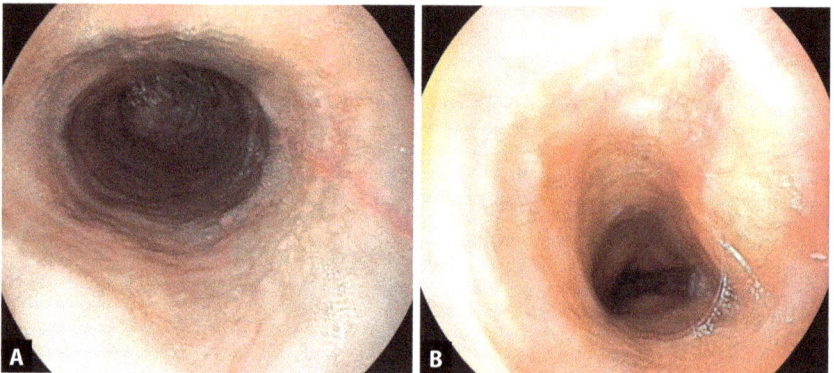

Figs. 2A and B: Eosinophilic esophagitis—(mild A) and (severe B).

understood but food allergy has been implicated as a primary contribution, on endoscopy there is not much difference between it and reflux esophagitis **(Figs. 1 and 2)**.[3]

The rate of incidence of EOE is different in different places. EOE annual incidence rates vary between 0 and 1 and 1.2 per 10,000 in several studies, with EOE representing the second most common cause of chronic esophagitis.[4]

The new consensus criteria published in 2011 emphasized that EOE is an antigen-driven, immune-triggered disease that requires adequate treatment with PPI therapy prior to finding >15 eosinophils high-power field (HPF; peak value) in the esophagus. These updated criteria also established the existence of PPI-responsive esophageal eosinophilia, but its relationship (in terms of etiology) to PPI-resistant esophageal eosinophilia (classic EOE) has not been established.[5]

It has been shown that dietary therapy frequently improves symptoms and reduces the number of eosinophils in esophageal biopsies of patients with primary EOE (allergic or nonallergic subtypes).

A diet consisting of an amino acid-based formula, termed an alimental diet, or avoidance of the most common allergenic foods (cow's milk, soy, wheat, egg, peanut/tree nuts, and seafood/shellfish), termed the six-food elimination diet (SFED), is advocated.[6]

Eosinophilic esophagitis occurs due to allergy to food material or acid reflux. There is inflammation of esophageal wall by eosinophils. The most common symptoms of EOE are dysphagia.

Lymphocytic Esophagitis

Lymphocytic esophagitis is a rare esophageal condition. The inner lining of the wall of esophagus is infiltrated with lymphocytes. Lymphocytic esophagitis may be related to GERD.

Infectious Esophagitis

Infectious esophagitis is caused by fungal, viral, or bacterial infection. It is quite uncommon. It is seen in people with poor immune function, i.e., human immunodeficiency virus (HIV).

Drug-induced Esophagitis

Some medicines which we take as a routine for pain, infection, hypertension, and weak bones can cause drug-induced esophagitis. Common medicines are:
- Pain relieving medicines such as aspirin and ibuprofen
- Antibiotics—tetracycline and doxycycline
- Quinidine used for heart problems
- Potassium chloride.

REFERENCES

1. Ronkainen J, Aro P, Storkskrubb T, Johansson SE, Lind T, Bolling-Sternevald E, et al. High prevalence of gastroesophageal reflux symptoms and esophagitis with or without symptoms in general Swedish population: A Kalixanda study report. Scand J Gastroenterol. 2005;40:275-85.
2. Danisa MC, Hachem C. Gastroesophageal reflux disease (GERD). Mo Med. 2018:115(3): 214-8.
3. Feldman M, Friedman LS, Brandt LJ. Sleisenger and Fordtran's book Gastrointestinal and Liver Disease, 10th edition. Philadelphia: Saunders Elsevier; 2016. pp. 456.
4. Feldman M, Friedman LS, Brandt LJ. Sleisenger and Fordtran's book Gastrointestinal and Liver Disease, 10th edition. Philadelphia: Saunders Elsevier; 2016. pp. 462.
5. Feldman M, Friedman LS, Brandt LJ. Sleisenger and Fordtran's book Gastrointestinal and Liver Disease, 10th edition. Philadelphia: Saunders Elsevier; 2016. pp. 457.
6. Kagalwala AF, Sentongo PA, Ritz S, Hess T, Nelson SP, Emerick KM, et al. Effect of six-food elimination diet on clinical and histological outcomes in eosinophilic esophagitis. Clin Gastroenterol Hepatol. 2006;4:1097-102.

CHAPTER 12

Prognosis

You can believe the diagnosis, not the prognosis.

–Deepak Chopra

Gastroesophageal reflux disease (GERD) is one of the most common problems world over. The prognosis of GERD is very good with treatment. The lifestyle changes and common over-the-counter (OTC) medicines can make a life easy and trouble free. If one concentrates on diet and identifies trigger foods then eliminations of food items may eliminate symptoms even without treatment.

Similarly, like trigger foods, one can identify medicines causing symptoms due to lax lower esophagus sphincter (LES) and can also be eliminated from regular use leading to complete relief.

Reducing meal size and avoiding fats, carminatives, and chocolate reduce reflux frequency by decreasing episodes of transient LES relaxations (TLESRs), as well as lowering LES pressure. In an evidence-based review, studies of smoking, alcohol, chocolate, fatty foods, and citrus products had some physiologic data that their intake can adversely affect symptoms or promote reflux on esophageal pH tests. Only elevation of the head of the bed, left lateral decubitus positioning, and weight loss were associated with GERD improvement in case-controlled studies.[1]

Alcohol and smoking are known risk factors for GERD and if stopped can give a major relief in symptoms and also reduce the chances of developing complications such as Barrett's esophagus.

In two large-randomized studies, open and laparoscopic anti-reflux surgery was not found to be superior to proton pump inhibitor (PPI) therapy, especially when dose titration was permitted.[2]

■ REFERENCES

1. Keltenbach T, Crockett S, Gerson LB. Are lifestyle measures effective in patients with gastroesophageal reflux disease? An evidence-based approach. Arch Intern Med. 2006;166:965-71.
2. Galmiche JP, Hatebakk JH, Attwood S, Ell C, Fiocca R, Eklund S, et al. Laparoscopic antireflux surgery esomeprazole treatment for chronic GERD. The LOTUS randomized clinical trial. JAMA. 2011;305:1969-77.

CHAPTER 13

Management of Gastroesophageal Reflux Disease

No disease that can be treated by diet should be treated with other means.
−Moses Maimonides (Jewish Philosopher)

Gastroesophageal reflux disease (GERD) is a common problem and is gradually increasing all over the globe. The reason for increasing incidence probably and most commonly is our faulty lifestyle. Smoking, alcohol, fatty food, stress, anger, overwork, and spicy food are common risk factors of today's life.

MODALITIES OF TREATMENT OF GASTROESOPHAGEAL REFLUX DISEASE

Following are the modalities of treatment of GERD.

Lifestyle Changes

Lifestyle if unhealthy must be made healthy and certain other changes to be advised in relation to GERD. In case of uncomplicated GERD, the first line of treatment should be lifestyle changes, but these should be taken seriously by patients. Clinician must have first session with the patient only about knowing his or her lifestyle and should find out the lacunae in lifestyle which require changes. One has to give the patient in writing about what lifestyle changes are required. These are:

- Elevate head end of bed, about 9".
- Maintain healthy weight.
- Stop smoking.
- Stop alcohol consumption.
- Go to bed 3 hours after a meal.
- Avoid foods that start reflux such as fatty foods, coffee, and spicy foods.
- Avoid large meals and take small frequent meals.
- Try to sleep on your left side.
- Avoid medicines which stimulate GERD symptoms, i.e., calcium channel blockers, sleeping pills, and sedatives such as benzodiazepines, theophylline, and nitrates.

Lifestyle changes definitely help persons with GERD, but weight loss and avoiding recumbency are the only two factors which have evidences by many researchers.

Two large prospective populations-based cohort studies showed that weight reduction does definitely decrease reflux symptoms.[1,2]

Antacids

Antacids neutralize acid in stomach. Antacids can give relief in symptoms of mild GERD but cannot heal the esophageal inflammation or erosion. These are only used when a person has occasional heartburn. For best results, antacids should be taken about an hour after a meal. Antacids can treat you symptomatically but cannot cure. Calcium carbonate (chalk) is very commonly used antacid. It is quite effective. Effervescent antacids and neutralizes stomach acid. Antacids come in two forms (1) liquid and (2) tablet. Tablets are chewable. Liquid antacids act quickly to release heartburn. Liquid antacids act faster than chewable tablet antacids. Alginic acid products are found to be much more effective than other antacids. Usually, they contains sodium alginate, sodium bicarbonate, and calcium carbonate. It comes as liquid as well as tablet.

Side Effects of Antacids

If antacids are taken daily, then this may cause:
- Headache
- Constipation
- Diarrhea
- Gas or flatulence
- Pain in abdomen
- Nausea
- Vomiting
- Osteoporosis
- Kidney stones and kidney damage
- Heart rhythm abnormalities

Antacids provide immediate relief from heartburn but they cannot heal the injury caused by acid on esophageal mucosa. Antacids are commonly used as they are available easily over the counter without doctor's prescription. Antacids neutralize the acid.

Histamine-2 Receptor Antagonists

These histamine-2 receptor antagonists (H2RAs) are available over the counter and you can purchase without having a doctor's prescription. They decrease acid production in stomach specially postprandial acid secretion. Common H2RAs (also called H2 blockers) are cimetidine, ranitidine, famotidine, and nizatidine. They are more effective than any antacid in treating symptoms of GERD. A course of 8 weeks with H2RA can heal almost half the cases of GERD (50%).

Rarely, H2RAs can cause cytopenias, gynecomastia, liver function test disturbances, and antiandrogenic effects.

Following are some examples of H2RAs:
- Cimetidine
- Ranitidine
- Famotidine
- Nizatidine

Mechanism Action

Acid is secreted by parietal cells of gastric mucosa; Histamine-2 receptors are situated on the surface of parietal cells. These H2RAs are in a competition with histamine at H_2-receptors and H_2-receptors take H2RAs instead of histamine so get blocked by H2RAs so they function as antagonists. When after a meal, parietal cells release histamine to combine with H_2-receptor on parietal cells of stomach and release acid but H2RAs are blocking the H_2-receptors and so by blocking the histamine receptor and thus histamine stimulations of parietal cell acid secretion, H2RAs suppress both stimulated and basal gastric acid secretion induced by histamine.[3]

To get proper effect in GERD, H2RAs should be given in two divided doses for at least 8 weeks and then if required on single dose maintenance therapy.

Healing rates of esophagitis with H2RAs are good but not as good as with Proton pump inhibitors (PPIs).

Notes:
- 1828—Charles Millard in Paris noticed the first case of esophagitis in child.
- 1879—Heinrich Quincke reported that ulceration in the esophagus was due to gastroesophageal reflux.
- 1906—Tilston described the typical symptoms of esophagitis.

The H2RAs side effects are minor, mild, and reversible.

> Notes:
> - Some patients develop tolerance to H2RAs after few weeks use in GERD.
> - Cimetidine may cause gynecomastia after a long-term use.

PROTON PUMP INHIBITORS

- PPIs are more effective than H2RAs in treating symptoms of GERD.
- PPIs after a course of 8 weeks treatment have better healing in erosive esophagitis than H2RAs.

Common PPIs are:
- Omeprazole and lansoprazole
- Esomeprazole and pantoprazole
- Rabeprazole and dexlansoprazole

Some researchers have believed that esomeprazole 40 mg is best at treating GERD.

- PPIs block the major pathways of gastric acid production and they do this better than H2RAs.
- A single study showed that esomeprazole at doses of 20 mg and 40 mg is more effective than 20 mg once a day in both healing and symptoms resolutions in GERD patients with reflux esophagitis, with a tolerability profile comparable to that of omeprazole. A randomized controlled treatment compared esomeprazole 40 mg to lansoprazole 30 mg. Esomeprazole was superior in healing and symptom control, with highest results in more severe degrees of esophagitis.[4]

Proton pump inhibitors block the gastric H,K-ATPase, inhibiting gastric acid secretion.[5] Because of the H,K-ATPase is the final step of acid secretion, an inhibitor of this enzyme is more effective than receptor antagonists in suppressing gastric acid secretion.[6]

The PPIs after 8 weeks treatment have better rate of healing than H2RAs in esophagitis in GERD. It is better to use PPI twice a day before meals for 8 weeks to seek best results of PPIs in GERD.

Esomeprazole is found to have better effect than omeprazole and lansoprazole in esophagitis of GERD but omeprazole is better for nighttime acid suppression. PPIs are very safe medicines and have only minimal side effects such as headache and diarrhea that is why they are in maximum use in GERD.

Baclofen

It is used to treat as a muscle relaxant in muscle spasm. It is not a pain killer but relieves pain by relaxing the muscle in spasm. It gives some relief to some patients of GERD.

Prokinates

Some prokinates are following:
- Cisapride
- Metoclopramide
- Domperidone
- Mosapride
- Itopride
- Renzapride

FAILURE OF GASTRO-ESOPHAGEAL REFLUX DISEASE MEDICAL TREATMENT

The GERD patients with classical symptoms should be treated with acid reducing drugs such as H2RAs and PPIs for at least 4 weeks, if the response of these drugs is partial, the treatment should be continued for 8 weeks, even in double dose if required. If there is no improvement with this treatment, patient should undergo upper gastrointestinal (GI) endoscopy. If a patient does not show response in 3 months, then it should be taken as the patient is suffering with some other disease and investigations should be concentrated on that line.

Do not prescribe H2RAs or PPIs indefinitely as the patient may develop serious complications of GERD.

STEP-UP AND STEP-DOWN TREATMENT

Usually, the patient starts treating his/her symptoms of GERD by antacids and when he does not get relief he goes to a clinician. If clinician treats the patient with H2RAs then should be treated for 2 weeks and if the response is partial, patient should be shifted to PPIs. If a patient is treated with PPIs for 4–8 weeks and shows a good response then one can shift to H2RAs.

TREATMENT OF PREGNANT PATIENT

The symptoms of GERD in pregnancy are due to two reasons:
1. Hormonal influence
2. Mechanical pressure on stomach by enlarging uterus

Initially, a pregnant patient should be treated with lifestyle alterations and antacids. If this gives good response then this treatment should be continued, if not then change to H2RAs which are found safe during pregnancy. If H2RAs do not give sufficient response then PPIs to be used, but with extreme precautions.

ELDERLY PATIENTS WITH GASTROESOPHAGEAL REFLUX DISEASE

These patients should first be checked with upper GI endoscopy as at this age malignancy is not rare. H2RAs and even PPIs can be considered, but only after doing upper GI endoscopy.

NONSPECIFIC TREATMENT OF GASTROESOPHAGEAL REFLUX DISEASE

Some demulcents have been tried by people to reduce the irritation of esophagus lining due to acid reflux in GERD with success. These demulcents give some relief by soothing the injured and inflamed mucus membrane caused by acid. They form a protective film over inflamed surface of esophageal mucosa. Licorice is used as a demulcent by many individuals and with reasonable relief, but the relief occurs only for an hour or so.

CHRONIC DRUG THERAPY FOR GASTROESOPHAGEAL REFLUX DISEASE

The PPIs are better than H2RAs, it is shown by various studies but still the problem of recurrence is with both groups of medicines. After a long treatment of severe esophagitis due to GERD, the relapses are more with H2RAs than PPIs, so in cases of severe esophagitis the treatment should be given as a maintenance therapy when relapse of symptoms starts. It is recommended that maintenance therapy should be at half dose for once a day, or twice a day.

Currently, acid suppressive therapy with PPIs has proved to be the first line of treatment.[7] PPIs are used as well as for healing erosions.[8] Although symptomatic relief and acute healing of esophageal lesions can be achieved by short-term PPI treatments in up to 75% of patients with nonerosive reflux disease (NERD) and up to 90% of patients with erosive reflux disease (ERD), patients experience relapse within 6 months–1 year after termination of initial treatments. Therefore, long-term continuous maintenance treatment with PPIs is required for the majority of patients with GERD to adequately control symptoms and to heal mucosal lesions.[9,10]

HOME REMEDIES FOR IMMEDIATE RELIEF IN ACID REFLUX

- Cold milk
- Chewing gum
- Egg white
- Ginger
- Curd
- Mint
- Coconut
- Tulsi leaves
- Oats
- Aloe Vera Juice
- Butter Milk
- Banana
- Raw Almond
- Pineapple juice
- Jaggery
- Watermelon Juice

London Gastroenterology Centre recommends what to eat and what not to eat if you have acid reflux, they recommend that if you are suffering with acid reflux then avoid coffee, chocolate, fizzy drinks, spicy fatty food, citrus fruits, and alcohol instead take herbal tea, fresh fruits, rice cakes, bread, banana, pears, lean meat and fish.

HEALING OF ESOPHAGEAL MUCOSAL ACID INJURY

Mucosa heals faster than skin. Acid damage to the mucosa of esophagus due to acid reflux or esophagitis can heal completely, one has to eat a soft and bland diet in small quantity to help the mucosa to heal faster. Avoid alcohol and smoking. GERD should be treated as soon as it is diagnosed as the acid reflux of GERD from stomach causes esophageal mucosa damage but it heals well with treatment but if it is neglected than permanent damage can occur which may lead to Barrett's esophagus.

SURGICAL TREATMENT OF GASTROESOPHAGEAL REFLUX DISEASE

Antireflux surgery (ARS) is widely accepted as a way of treatment when medical treatment fails or disease becomes resistant to medical treatment. The most common surgical procedure is Nissen's fundoplication. It is taken as a gold standard of surgical treatment of GERD.

It is a wraparound procedure of stomach around the lowest part of esophagus. It strengthens lower esophageal sphincter (LES) to avoid acid reflux.

Most of the patients suffering with GERD can manage satisfactorily with lifestyle alterations and acid reducing drugs, but those who are suffering in spite of this management can either continue suffering like this and develop serious complications such as Barrett's esophagus and carcinoma of esophagus or go for Nissen's fundoplication and live life better.

Cases refractory to medical therapy should be treated by surgical intervention.

Nissen's Fundoplication

This is the best available surgical procedure for GERD as it is a time tested procedure.

Before this procedure of ARS, following must be done:
- Upper GI endoscopy
- Barium esophagogram
- Esophageal manometry
- 24-hour esophageal pH testing

These tests are done before the surgical procedure is planned to exclude esophageal stricture, carcinoma of esophagus, hiatus hernia, achalasia, etc. Careful testing will result in modification of the original operation or an alternative diagnosis in approximately 30% of patients.[11]

Although widely quoted in the study of DeMeester et al.,[12] which demonstrated a positive outcome for 91% of patients undergoing open Nissen's fundoplication, extrapolated a 10-year outcome through an actual analysis with a series that reported an average follow-up of 45 months.

Antireflux surgery may be open or laparoscopic. There is clear evidence for the benefits of laparoscopic ARS (LARS). Many different LARS techniques are available.[13] They include fundoplication, anterior 180° wrap; Toupet fundoplication, a posterior 220° wrap; and Nissen's fundoplication, a total posterior 360° wrap.[14]

Nissen's fundoplication can be done by open or laparoscopic techniques. Most common ARS performed in the United States is the Laparoscopic Nissen's fundoplication.[15-19] Indications of Nissen's fundoplication or ARS are:
- Failed medical treatment
- Repeated aspiration pneumonia due to GERD
- Patient who does not want to take medical therapy for long.
- Cannot continue medical therapy due to side effects of medicines.

ENDOSCOPIC TREATMENT PROCEDURES FOR GASTROESOPHAGEAL REFLUX DISEASE

Now a days various endoscopic antireflux procedures are developed to treat GERD. All these methods are not very common at present. These procedures are:
- Radiofrequency ablation (RFA)
- Transoral incisionless fundoplication (TIF)
- Medigus ultrasonic surgical endostapler (MUSE)
- Antireflux mucosectomy (ARMS).

Radiofrequency Ablation

Stretta system (Mederi Therapeutics, USA) applied radiofrequency to LES and gastric cardia in relation to Z line. It gives low-frequency heat to reshape LES with additional strength so it should act normally **(Fig. 1)**.

Transoral Incisionless Fundoplication

In this procedure, endoscopically gastric fundus is wrapped around lower esophagus. Plastic fasteners are used which are accepted by the body **(Fig. 2)**.

Medigus Ultrasonic Surgical Endostapler

It is an incisionless fundoplication. Here, a modified endoscope and endostapler is used

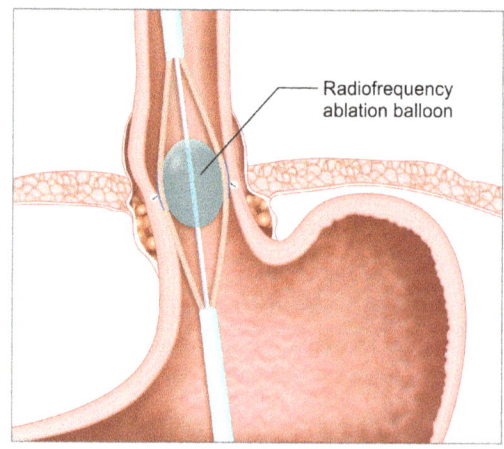

Fig. 1: Radiofrequency ablation balloon.

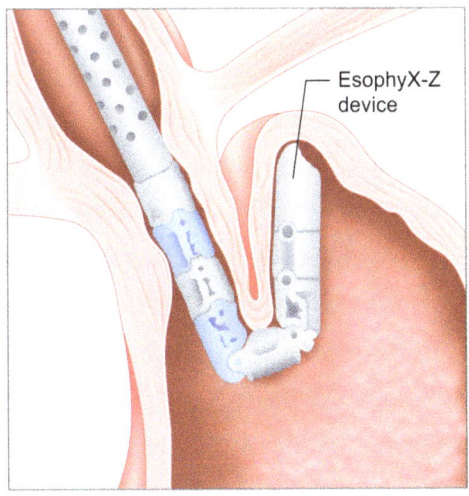

Fig. 2: Transoral incisionless fundoplication.

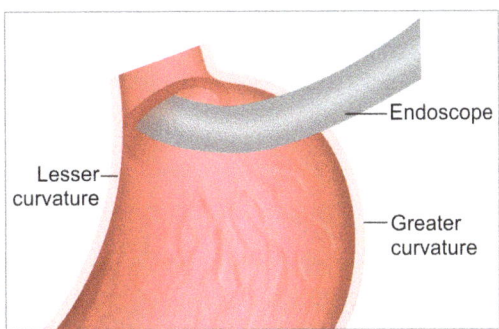

Fig. 4: Antireflux mucosectomy.

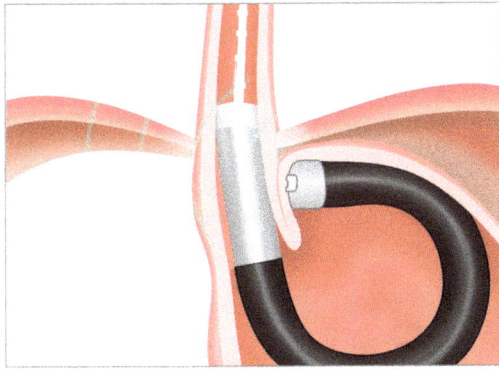

Fig. 3: Medigus ultrasonic surgical endostapler.

with a camera and ultrasound probe. It staples the gastric fundus with esophagus 3 cm proximal to gastroesophageal junction. This procedure requires more time and more study to prove the efficacy of the procedure **(Fig. 3)**.

Antireflux Mucosectomy

In this procedure, endoscopic resection of mucosa over gastroesophageal junction is done. The wound so created gradually heals and contracts, which reduces the gastroesophageal reflux **(Fig. 4)**.

REFERENCES

1. Jacobson BC, Somers SC, Fuchs CS, Kelly CP, Camargo CA Jr. Body-mass index and symptoms of gastroesophageal reflux in women. N Engl J Med. 2006;354(22):2340-8.
2. Ness-Jensen E, Lindam A, Lagergren J, Hveem K. Weight loss and reduction in gastroesophageal reflux. A prospective population-based cohort study: the HUNT study. Am J Gastroenterol. 2013;108(3):376-82.
3. Macfarlane B. Management of gastroesophageal reflux disease in adults: a pharmacist's perspective. Integer Pharm Res Pract. 2018;7:4-52.
4. UMAS GERD Guideline, September, 2013.
5. Shin JM, Sachs G. Pharmacology of proton pump inhibitors. Curr Gastroenterol Rep. 2008;10(6):528-34.
6. Fellenius E, Berglinoth T, Sachs G, Olbe L, Elander B, Sjöstrand SE, et al. Substituted benzimidazoles inhibit gastric acid secretion by blocking (H+, K+) ATPase. Nature. 1981;290:159-61.
7. Katz PO, Gerson LB, Vela MF. Guidelines for the diagnosis and management of gastroesophageal reflux disease. Am J Gastroenterol. 2013;108:308-28.
8. Van Pinxteren B, Numans MB, Bonis PA, Lau J, Numans ME. Short-term treatment with proton pump inhibitors, H_2-receptor antagonists and prokinetics for gastro-oesophageal reflux disease-like symptoms and endoscopy negative reflux disease. Cochrane Database Syst Rev. 2013;2013(5):CD002095.

9. Dean BB, Gano ADJD, Knight K, Ofman JJ, Fass R. Effectiveness of proton pump inhibitors in nonerosive reflux disease. Clin Gastroenterol Hepatol. 2004;2(8):656-64.
10. Kang SJ, Jung HK, Tac CH, Kim SY, Lee KJ. On-demand versus continuous maintenance and treatment of gastroesophageal reflux disease with proton pump inhibitors: a systemic review and meta-analysis. J Neurogastroenterol Motil. 2022;28(1):5-14.
11. Chan WW, Haroian LR, Gyuwali GP. Value of preoperative esophageal function studies before laparoscopic antireflux surgery. Surg Endosc. 2011;25:2950-5.
12. DeMeester TR, Bonavina L, Albartucci M. Nissen fundoplication for gastroesophageal reflux disease: evaluation of primary, repair in 100 consecutive patients. Ann Surg. 1986;204(1):9-20.
13. Seevas K, Bitar K, Siccardi MA. Nissen fundoplication. Treasure Island (FL): StatPearls Publishing; 2023.
14. Frazzoni M, Piccoli M, Conigliaro R, Frazzoni L, Metott G. Laparoscopic fundoplication for gasteroesophageal reflux disease. World J Gastroenterol. 2014;20(39):14272-9.
15. Linzberger N, Berdah SV, Orsoni P, Faucher D, Grimand JC, Picaud R. Laparoscopic posterior fundoplication in gastroesophageal reflux: Mid-term result. Ann Chir. 2001;126(2):143-7.
16. Mardam J, Lundell L, Engtrom C. Total or posterior partial fundoplication in the treatment of GERD: results of a randomized trial after 2 decades of follow-up. Am Surg. 2011;253(5):875-8.
17. Du X, Wu JM, Hu ZW, Wang F, Wang ZG, Zhang C, et al. Laparoscopic Nissen (total) versus anterior 180 degree fundoplication for gastro-esophageal reflux disease: A meta-analysis and systematic review. Medicine (Baltimore). 2017;96(37):e8085.
18. Du X, Hu Z, Yan C, Zhang C, Wang Z, Wu J. A meta-analysis of long follow-up outcomes of laparoscopic Nissan (total) versus Toupe (270) fundoplication for gastro-esophageal reflux disease based on randomized controlled trials in adults. BMC Gastroenterol. 2016;16(1):88.
19. Broeders JA, Mauritz FA, Ahmed Ali U, Draouisma WA, Ruurda JP, Gooszen HG, et al. Systematic review and meta-analysis of laparoscopic Nissen (posterior total) versus Toupet (posterior partial) fundoplication for gastro-oesophageal reflux disease. Br J Surg. 2010;97(9):1318-30.

CHAPTER 14

Barrett's Esophagus

I don't believe in hope. I believe in action, if I am an apostle of anything: there are always going to be complications, but to a large degree, everything is in your hand.
—Kerry James Marshall

Barrett's esophagus (BE) is a condition in which an abnormal columnar epithelium that is predisposed to malignancy replaces the stratified squamous epithelium that normally lines the distal esophagus.[1] BE is diagnosed by a history of gastroesophageal reflux disease (GERD) especially chronic, upper gastrointestinal (GI) endoscopy, and endoscopic biopsy of the mucosa at gastroesophageal junction site. Histopathology shows the metaplasia of squamous epithelium to columnar epithelium.

The prevalence of BE is between 1.6 and 6.8% in West.[2,3] The reported rates of BE ranged from 2.6 to 23% in Indian patients with GERD symptom.[4]

When the columnar epithelium replaces squamous epithelium of esophagus >3 cm in length at the lower part of esophagus it is called as "short-segment BE". According to some researches, there may be increased incidence of development of malignancy in short-segment BE. BE mucosa contains cells of different grades of dysplasia from nondysplasia to cancer.

Endoscopic resection or radiofrequency may be advised for dysplasia and early adenocarcinoma.[5]

Columnar-lined esophagus (Barrett's) esophagus was named-after by Norman Rupert Barrett (1903–1979) in 1950.[6]

The squamocolumnar junction draws up by scar tissue into the mediastinum.[7,8] Some researchers did not agree with this statement.[9,10]

According to recent guidelines in high-grade dysplasia (HGD), the risk of developing cancer might be at 10% per patient year or greater.[11]

Long-segment BE is found in 3–5% whereas 10–20% have short-segment BE.[12] However, a number of large studies published since 2011 have suggested that the cancer risk for such patients is even lower, in the range of 0.12–0.33% per year.[13]

WHY BARRETT'S ESOPHAGUS BECOMES MALIGNANT?

Recently, it has been proposed that cells also might need to acquire two additional physiological features to become malignant. First, they must reprogram their energy metabolism in order to support the continuous proliferation required of tumor cells. Second, they must evade destruction by immune cells, including T and B lymphocytes, macrophages, and natural killer cells.[14]

Patients of BE have risk of developing adenocarcinoma of esophagus (AE) in <1% patients.

Barrett's esophagus cannot be diagnosed only by history and proton pump inhibitor (PPI) trial treatment test. BE is diagnosed by upper gastrointestinal endoscopy and histopathology.

We require highly advanced and sensitive endoscopic methods to diagnose early esophageal dysplasia or mucosal changes in esophagus to avoid development of AE.

Latest endoscopic techniques to treat advanced esophageal dysplasia and carcinoma of esophagus are very effective.

FACTORS RESPONSIBLE FOR BARRETT'S ESOPHAGUS IN GERD

- Low pressure at lower esophageal sphincter (LES)
- Weak esophageal peristalsis
- Impaired esophagogastric junction
- Hyperacid secretion by gastric mucosa
- Bile reflux
- Diminished secretion of EGF (epidermal growth factor)

The EGF is a salivary protein which helps in regeneration of cells.

Note: Very little is known about the tumor-promoting effects on esophageal cells in BE. Aneuploidy has been proposed as a biomarker for neoplastic progression in BE.[15]

PATHOGENESIS OF BARRETT'S ESOPHAGUS

The GERD exposes lower esophageal mucosa to acid and when chronic, it leads to esophagitis which results in BE by replacing stratified squamous epithelium with gastric columnar epithelium. BE develops by reprogramming of cells of lower esophagus to produce metaplasia in GERD.

Nitrate and Barrett's Esophagus

Spinach, beetroot, potatoes, cabbage, lettuce, radish, and some other leafy vegetables and fruits contain higher amount of nitrates. Processed nonvegetarian foods are rich in nitrates such as sausages, salami, and bacon.

American gastroenterological societies consider the specialized epithelium with goblet cells a requirement for the diagnosis of BE. British guidelines consider the possibility of including BE with gastric metaplasia.

Note: Most patients of BE will not develop cancer. In some patients, however, a precancerous change in the tissue, called dysplasia, will develop that precancerous changes are more likely to develop into esophageal cancer.
–American Society for Gastrointestinal Endoscopy

When nitrates present in food, mix with gastric juice acid they convert into nitrous acid, nitroso compounds, and nitric oxide. These products react with N-nitrosatable compounds, they form N-nitroso compounds which are potentially carcinogenic. Antioxidants such as vitamin C can help to reduce its effects of nitrates.

Prague Classification of Barrett's Esophagus

It was given by International Working Group for the Classification of Oesophagitis (IWGCO) in 2004.[16]

This classification uses "C" value for circumferential factor and "M" value for maximum length (tongue like lesion).

DIAGNOSIS

Barrett's esophagus is diagnosed with an upper gastrointestinal endoscopy and mucosal biopsy.

Histology shows the difference between normal and even early BE **(Figs. 1 and 2)**.

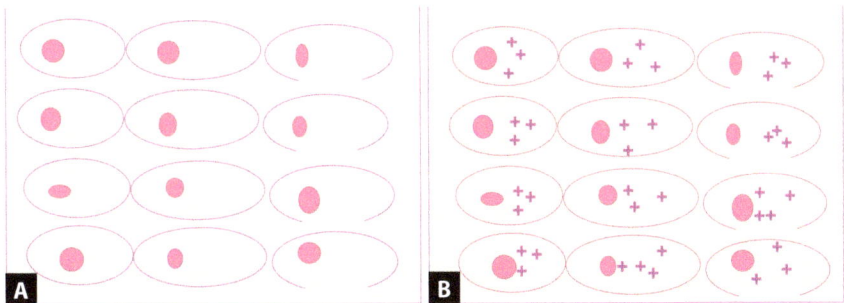

Figs. 1A and B: (A) Normal esophageal mucosa; (B) Barrett's esophageal mucosa, diagrammatically.

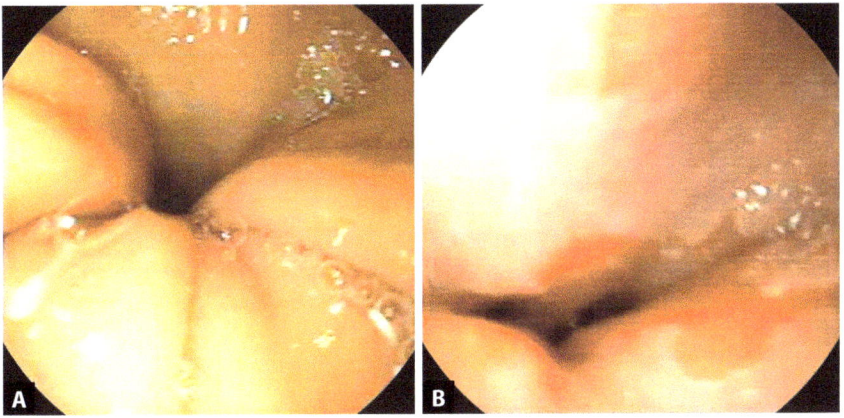

Figs. 2A and B: (A) Normal esophageal mucosa on endoscopy; (B) Barrett's esophageal mucosa on endoscopy.

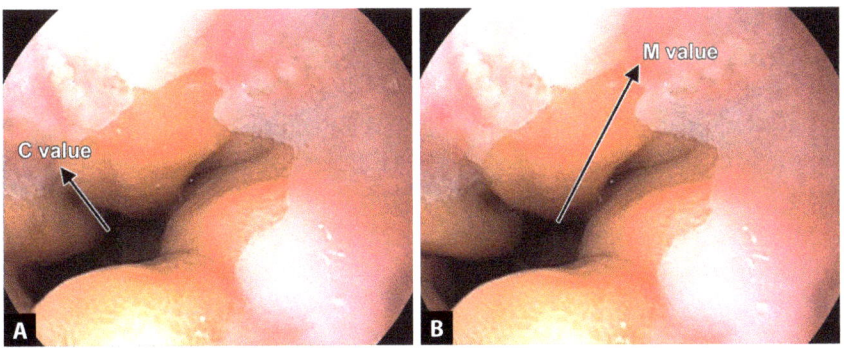

Figs. 3A and B: (A) C value as per Prague classification; (B) M value as per Prague classification of Barrett's esophagus.

The Prague classification of BE is to report the extent of BE and there will be uniformity in different centers reporting BE and thus confusion will be avoided **(Figs. 3A and B)**.

There are factors responsible for conversion of BE to AE. BE is a premalignant condition as it has high cellular growth rate, low death rate, and increased diploid and aneuploid cells compared to normal epithelium.[17,18]

These factors are responsible for the malignant transformation which is observed in the progression of BE.[19]

Dysplasia in Barrett's Esophagus

Dysplasia indicates presence of abnormal cells in BE, other than columnar cells. It may be (1) mild dysplasia or (2) severe dysplasia. Mild dysplasia has very little changes and sometimes it is difficult to differentiate the BE cells from dysplastic cells with many changes in cells. Severe dysplasia is the later stage of transformation to malignancy.

Dysplasia includes nuclear changes, loss of cytoplasmic maturation, and crowding of tubules and villiform surfaces.[20]

MANAGEMENT OF BARRETT'S ESOPHAGUS

- Lifestyle changes
- Proton pump inhibitor (PPIs)
- Other methods of treatment:
  - Endoscopic ablative therapy by laser, radiofrequency energy ablation (REA), electrocoagulation, etc.
  - Cryotherapy
  - Photochemical energy
  - Photodynamic therapy (PDT)
  - Endoscopic mucosal resection (EMR)

Lifestyle Changes

Lifestyle changes which are effective include:
- Stopping smoking
- Stopping alcohol
- Eating small and frequent meals
- Avoid symptoms triggering foods such as coffee, chocolate, spicy and fatty foods.

Lifestyle alterations much be tried even when treatment of BE is on.

Proton Pump Inhibitor (PPI)

The PPIs are the required drugs to treat BE.

Barrett's esophagus is one of the complications of GERD. Acid suppression with PPIs has become the mainstay of treatment of patients with BE.[21]

Irrespective of doses or length of treatment, healing of esophagitis is best and faster achieved with PPIs.[22]

The PPIs should be given for at least 8 weeks and then may be put on maintenance therapy.

Proton Pump Inhibitor Therapy and Adenocarcinoma of Esophagus

Cooper et al. published their study and told that, the incidence of adenocarcinoma was thought to be 1%,[23] but in 2001 Shaheen et al. reviewed the world literature and concluded that there was an inverse relationship between study size and cancer incidence.[24] They calculated that the real risk was 0.5%,[24] Jankowski et al. reviewed the British data and concluded that the British incidence was 0.98%.[25]

Other Methods

Radiofrequency Ablation

It is for only low-grade dysplasia (LGD) in BE. This destroys precancerous or dysplastic cells and they are gradually replaced by normal cells.

Cryoablation

This method is also used for LGDs. The extreme cold caused by liquid nitrogen or carbon dioxide destroys precancerous cells.

Endoscopic Mucosal Resection

Barrett's tissue is resected by a special equipment attached to the endoscope.

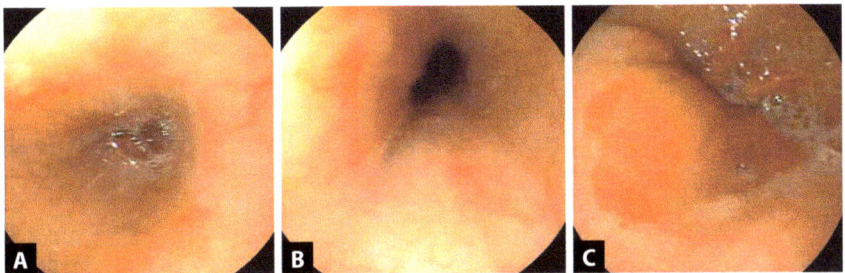

Figs. 4A to C: (A) Normal esophagus; (B) Inflamed esophagus; (C) Barrett's esophagus.

Esophagectomy

The part of esophagus having lesion is removed surgically and is replaced by the part of stomach or colon.

Endoscopic Surveillance for Barrett's Esophagus

Periodic endoscopic examination is required in BE as there is a possibility of cancer development. The surveillance may also take esophageal biopsy to see the status at cellular level. Patients with LGD in BE may need endoscopy about every 3 months. Frequency of endoscopic surveillance depends upon the severity of dysplasia.

Nonsteroidal Anti-inflammatory Drugs and Barrett's Esophagus

There is an indication by some researches that nonsteroidal anti-inflammatory drugs (NSAIDs) are helpful in colorectal and esophageal cancer.[26] G Morgan, writes NSAIDs be used for reversal of BE. Cox inhibition is thought to be the mechanism of colorectal prevention.[27]

Now, there are researches that point that NSAIDs may reduce the incidence of the risk of developing esophageal cancer.

> Current guidelines of BE patients recommend endoscopic surveillance at intervals of 3–5 years for patients without dysplasia, 6–12 months for those with low-grade dysplasia and every 3 months for HGD patients.[15,28]

Surveillance in patients with BE refers to the endoscopies performed at regular intervals with the goal to detect dysplasia and early cancer at a curable stage. Potentially, the early detection of esophageal adenocarcinoma can lead to decrease in mortality from this disease.[29]

Surveillance endoscopies are done in a patient of BE to detect dysplasia, its grading and a cancerous growth if developing. Early detection of most of the diseases leads to early treatment and the results also improve and same is true for BE. Surveillance endoscopies, therefore, are done in BE to improve prognosis.

Barrett's Esophagus (Figs. 4A to C)

Reflux esophagitis due to GERD is of two types or grades (1) mild and (2) erosive esophagitis.

Mild esophagitis shows only microscopic changes such as infiltration of mucosa of esophagus by granulocyte or eosinophils. It may look normal on endoscopy.

Erosive esophagitis can be diagnosed by endoscopy as the esophageal mucosa becomes inflamed, i.e., red, friable, and may also be having superficial ulcers. Erosive esophagitis may heal completely or become BE which becomes a matter of concern as it is a premalignant condition and may lead to AE.

Risk factor for BE includes:[30-33]
- Older than 50 years of age
- Male sex
- White race
- Family history of BE or esophageal adenocarcinoma.
- Prolonged reflux symptoms
- Smoking
- Obesity

It is advised that endoscopy and biopsy should not be done in a normal looking esophagus. If there is no dysplasia on histopathology after endoscopic biopsy of suspicious BE then endoscopy should be done between 3 and 5 years. If the dysplasia is of low-grade, endoscopic biopsy should be done between 6 and 12 months and if the dysplasia is of high grade then it should be done every 3 months.

Proton pump inhibitors should be given for GERD symptoms in morning and evening doses regularly and not intermittently. It has been advised that low-dose aspirin reduces cancer risk, but should be reserved for BE patients who have cardiovascular risk factors for which aspirin is indicated.[34]

> *Note:* Complications of GERD (i.e., BE and AE) are rare, but do exist; 10–15% with GERD will develop BE, and 1–10% of those with BE will develop adenocarcinoma over 10–20 years.
> –UMHS GERD Guidelines, September 2013

■ REFERENCES

1. Spechler SJ, Fitzgerald RC, Prasad GA, Wang KK. History, molecular mechanisms, and endoscopic treatment of Barrett's esophagus. Gastroenterology. 2010;138:854-69.
2. Rex DK, Cummings OW, Shaw M, Cumings MD, Wong RK, Vasudeva RS, et al. Screening for Barrett's esophagus in colonoscopy patients with and without heartburn. Gastroenterology. 2003;125:1670-7.
3. Roonkainen J, Aro P, Storskruble T, Johansson SE, Lind T, Bolling-Sternevald E, et al. Prevalence of Barrett's esophagus in the general population: an endoscopic study. Gastroenterology. 2005;129:1825-31.
4. Wani IR, Showkat HI, Bhargav DK, Samer M. Prevalence and risk factors for Barrett's esophagus in patients with GERD in Northern India; Do methylene blue-directed biopsies improve detection of Barrett's esophagus compared to conventional method? Middle East J Dig Dis. 2014;6(4):228-36.
5. Shaheen NJ, Falk GW, Iyer PG, Gerson LB; American College of Gastroenterology. ACG clinical guideline: diagnosis and management of Barrett's esophagus. Am J Gastroenterol. 2016;111(1):30-50;quiz 51.
6. Katz-Summercorn, Annalisic, Frankell, Alexander M, Fitz Gerald, Rebecca C. Chapter 4: Genetics and Biomarkers in Barrett's Esophagus and Esophageal Adenocarcinoma. In: Pleskow, Douglas P, Erim T (Eds). Barrett's Esophagus-Emerging Evidence for Improved Clinical Practice. United States: Academic Press Inc; 2016. pp. 57-60.
7. Barrett NR. Chronic peptic ulcer of the esophagus and esophagelis. Br J Surg. 1950;38(150):175-82.
8. DeMeester SR, De Meister TR. Columnar mucosa and intestinal metaplasia of the esophagus. Fifty years of controversy. Ann Surg. 2000;231(3):303-21.
9. Allison PR, Johnstone AS. The oesophagus lined with gastric mucous membrane. Thorax. 1953;8(2):87-101.
10. Allison PR. Peptic ulcer of the esophagus. Thorax. 1948;3(1):20-42.
11. Shahean NJ, Richter JE. Barrett's esophagus. Lancet. 2009;373(9666):850-61.
12. Feldman M, Friedman LS, Brandt LJ. Sleisenger and Fordtran's book Gastrointestinal and Liver Disease: Pathophysiology/Diagnosis/Management, 10th edition. Philadelphia, PA: Elsevier/Saunders; 2016. pp. 755.
13. Hvid-Jensen F, Pedersen L, Drewes AM, Sørensen HT, Funch-Jensen P. Incidence of adenocarcinoma among patients with Barrett's esophagus. N Engl J Med. 2011;365:1375-83.

14. Hanahan D, Weinberg RA. Hallmarks of cancer: The next generation. Cell. 2011; 144:646-74.
15. Spechler SJ, Sharma P, Souza RF, Inadomi JM, Shaheen NJ; American Gastroenterological Association. American Gastroenterological technical review on the management of Barrett's esophagus. Gastroenterology. 2011;140:e18-52.
16. Sharma P, Dent J, Armstrong D, Bergman JJ, Gossner L, Hoshihara Y, et al. The development and validation of an endoscopic grading system for Barrett's esophagus: The Prague C&M criteria. Gastroenterology. 2006;131:1392-9.
17. Chandrasoma P. Controversies of the cardiac mucosa and Barrett's oesophagus. Histopathology. 2005;46:361-73.
18. Reid BJ, Sanchez CA, Blount PL, Levine DS. Barrett's esophagus: cell cycle abnormalities in advancing stages of neoplastic progression. Gastroenterology. 1993;105:119-29.
19. Stawinski PM, Dziadkowiec KN, Kuo LA, Echavarria J, Satigran S. Barrett's esophagus: an updated review. Diagnostics. 2023;13(2): 321.
20. Feldman M, Friedman LS, Brandt LJ. Sleisenger and Fordtran's book Gastrointestinal and Liver Disease: Pathophysiology/Diagnosis/Management, 10th edition. Philadelphia, PA: Elsevier/Saunders; 2016. pp. 757.
21. Castell DO, Katzka DA. Barrett's esophagus. Continuing questions and controversy. Gastrointest Endosc. 1999;49:55-8.
22. Katzka DA, Castell DO. Successful elimination of reflux symptoms does not ensure adequate control of acid reflux in Barrett's esophagus. Am J Gastroenterol. 1994;89:989-91.
23. Dvewitz DJ, Sampliner RE, Garewal HS. The incidence of adenocarcinoma in Barrett's esophagus: a prospective study of 170 patients followed 4-8 years. Am J Gastroenterol 1997;92:212-5.
24. Shaheen NJ, Crosby MA, Bozymski EM, Sadler RS. Is there publication bias in the reporting of cancer risk in Barrett's esophagus. Gastroenterology. 2000;119:333-8.
25. Jankowski JA, Provenzale D, Moayyeddi P. Esophageal adenocarcinoma arising from Barrett's metaplasia has regional variations in the west. Gastroenterology. 2002;122: 588-91.
26. IARC. Non-steroidal anti-inflammatory drugs. IARC Handbooks of Cancer Prevention, Volume 1. Lyon: International Agency for Research on Cancer, 1997.
27. Funkhouser EM, Sharp GB. Aspirin and the reduced risk of esophageal cancer. Cancer. 1995;76:1116-9.
28. Wang KK, Sampliner RE. Updated guidelines 2008 for the diagnosis, surveillance, and therapy of Barrett's esophagus. Am J Gastroenterol. 2008;103:788-97.
29. Sharma P, Sidorenko EI. Are screening and surveillance for Barrett's oesophagus really worthwhile? Gut. 2005;54 Suppl 1(Suppl 1): i27-32.
30. Wo IM, Mendez C, Harrell S, Joubran R, Bressoud PF, McKinney WP. Clinical in impact of upper endoscopy in the management of patients with gastroesophageal reflux disease. Am J Gastroentrol. 2004;19:2311-6.
31. Lieberman DA, Qehlke M, Helfand M. Risk factors for Barrett's esophagus in community-based practice GORGE Consortium. Gastroenterology Outcomes Research Group in Endoscopy. Am J Gastroenterol. 1997;92:1293-7.
32. Shaheen NJ, Weinberg BS, Denberg TD, Chou R, Qaseem A, Shekelle P; Clinical Guidelines Committee of the American College of Physicians. Upper endoscopy for gastroesophageal reflux disease: best practice advise from the clinical guidelines committee of the American College of Physicians. Ann Intern Med. 2012;157:808-16.
33. ASGE Standards of Practice Committee; Evans JA, Early DS, Fukami N, Ben-Menachem T, Chandrasekhara V, Chathadi KV, et al. The role of endoscopy in Barrett's esophagus and other premalignant conditions of esophagus. Gastroentest Endosc. 2012;76:1087-94.
34. UMHS GERD Guidelines, September, 2013.

CHAPTER 15

Hiatus Hernia

Sometimes it is the complication, which just lies in our minds.
–Anamika Mishra

Hiatus hernia is a condition in which the upper portion of stomach is pushed above diaphragm through an opening or hiatus that's called hiatus hernia. Hiatus hernia can cause heartburn, acid regurgitation, chest or abdominal pain, dysphagia, and vomiting **(Figs. 1A to C)**.

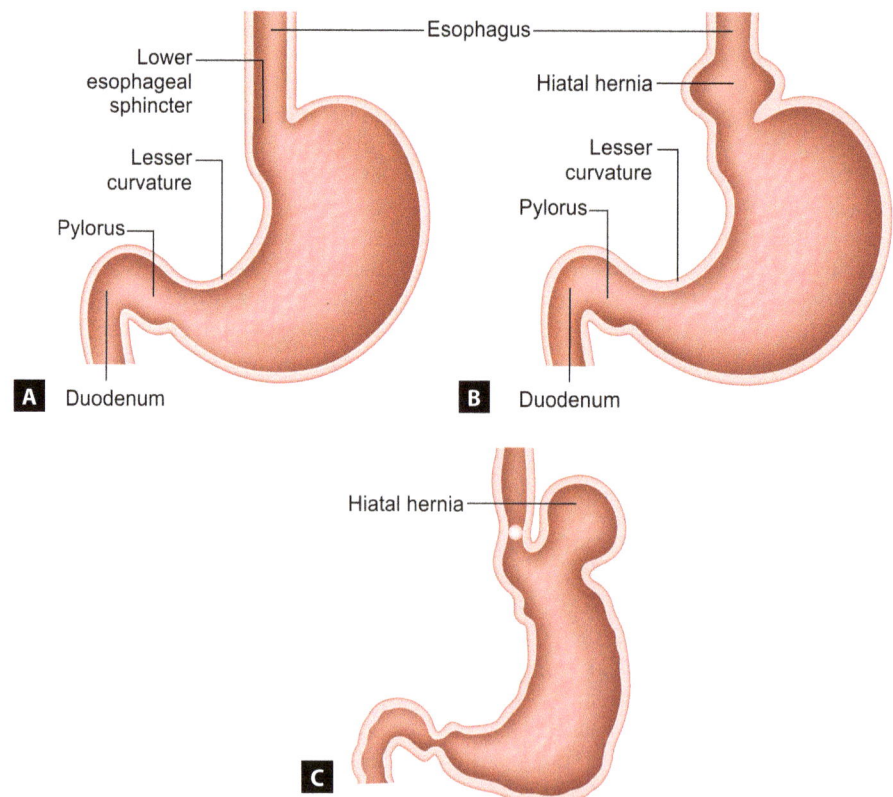

Figs. 1A to C: (A) Normal stomach; (B) Sliding hiatus hernia; (C) Paraesophageal hiatal hernia.

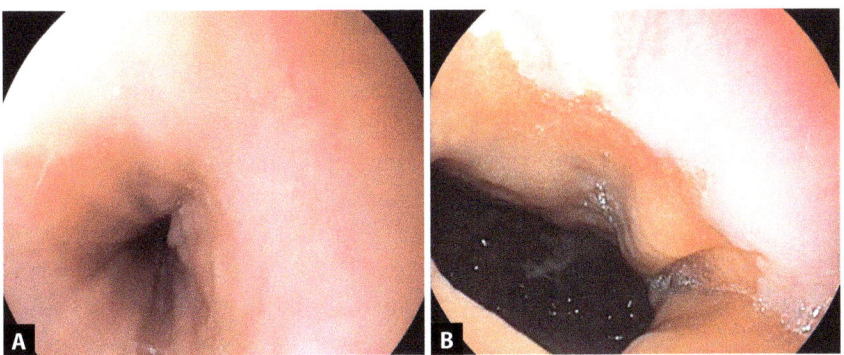

Figs. 2A and B: (A) Normal stomach; (B) Hiatus hernia.

Hiatus hernia increases the chances of gastroesophageal reflux disease (GERD) development through following factors:
- Hiatus hernia pushes lower esophageal sphincter (LES) up and so reduces the resting pressure of LES.
- LES is a high-pressure zone but due to upward displacement of LES due to hiatus hernia, the LES gets shortened.
- During straining, LES pressure increases but hiatus hernia eliminates it.
- Hiatus hernias increase the frequency of LES relaxations (LESRs).
- In hiatus hernias, the hernia sac acts as a pocket collecting acid from stomach (acid pocket) and this increases acid reflux.
- The gastric mucosal folds in acid pocket increase the tendency of reflux.
- LES also opens at lower pressure in hiatus hernias. Real mechanism of development of hiatus hernia is not clearly known but raised intra-abdominal pressure such as heavy weightlifting may cause hiatus hernia.

Acid pocket in a case of GERD is significantly responsible for acid reflux. In GERD with hiatus hernia, the acid pocket is bigger than in case of GERD without hiatus hernia and due to this reason in case of GERD with hiatus hernia, acid reflux is much more common and frequent **(Figs. 2A and B)**.

Hiatus hernia is a known risk factor for GERD. Hiatus hernias adversely affects the main acid reflux barrier, i.e., LES. Hiatus hernia influences LES and reduces its pressure leading to relaxation of LES, and opening of LES. Hiatus hernia leads to back leakage of acid in esophagus from stomach by following mechanisms:
- Relaxation of LES by reducing its contraction or pressure
- Transient LESR (TLESR) occurs quickly and recurrently by hiatus hernia.
- Esophageal clearance is delayed.
- Probably, the gastric contents in hiatus hernia sac leak back in esophagus when LES relaxes during swallowing of food.

TYPE OF HIATUS HERNIAS

There are four types of hiatus hernias.
1. *Type I*—sliding type. >90% hiatus hernias are of this type. It is usually associated with acid regurgitation or GERD.
2. *Type II*—paraesophageal hernia. Here, a part of esophagus escapes into chest, parallel to esophagus.
3. *Type III*—it is a combination of sliding and paraesophageal hernia.

4. *Type IV*—when along with stomach some other abdominal organ also herniates such as small intestine, colon, or spleen.

Type I and type III are commonly associated with GERD.

Patients with hiatus hernia may not be having GERD and some patients without much significant signs of hiatus hernia have advanced GERD. Hiatus hernias that are range (>3 m) and nonreducible (hernias in which the gastric rugal folds remain above the diaphragm between swallows) are especially prone to reflux.[1]

The hiatus hernia is the herniation of part of stomach through esophageal hiatus of the diaphragm. This happens when the esophageal hiatus is weak and lax. When the upper part of stomach escapes to the chest, the reflux of gastric contents with acid easily flows back to esophagus leading to GERD. Large hiatal hernias often require surgery.[2] Most important symptom is heartburn, followed by regurgitation. Regurgitation does not mean GERD as every patient of regurgitation in hiatus hernias does not have GERD. History of symptoms is important to diagnose hiatal hernia and with GERD. Physical examination in case of hiatal hernia and GERD is of not much importance.

Upper gastrointestinal endoscopy is the most important investigation tool to diagnose hiatus hernia with or without GERD. It is also important as it excludes serious esophageal diseases also, such as Barrett's esophagus and stricture of esophagus.

REFERENCES

1. Beaumort H, Bennink RJ, de Jong J, Boeckxstaens GE. The position of the acid pocket as a major risk factor for acidic reflux in healthy subjects and patients with GORD. Gut. 2010;59:441-51.
2. Kahrilas PJ, Kim HC, Pandrlfino JE. Approaches to the diagnosis and grading of hiatal hernia. Best Pract Res Clin Gastroenterol. 2008;22(4):601-16.

CHAPTER 16

Helicobacter pylori Infection

Life is really simple, but we insist on making it complicated.
—**Confucius**

Helicobacter pylori (Hp) has many strains which lead to various levels of pathological features. Patients who are infected with Hp usually get so in early life. Hp infection is more common in underdeveloped and developing countries than developed countries.

Helicobacter pylori infection, the most common chronic bacterial infection in the world, is linked to peptic ulcer disease (PUD) and gastric adenocarcinoma and is a key constituent of the human microbiome. Hp bacteria are having an abnormal quality of surviving in acidic medium. The flagella of the bacteria help them in their movement.

Dr Robin Warren discovered the spiral bacteria *Helicobacter pylori* in 1982. Hp is a gram-negative spiral bacterium. Hp causes gastritis and was well demonstrated by Dr Robin Warren and Dr Barry Marshall on themselves. It was proved later on that in association with gastritis Hp may also cause gastric ulcer (GU) and duodenal ulcer (DU) and can be well treated by antibiotics such as amoxicillin, clarithromycin, or metronidazole with a proton pump inhibitor (PPI). Marshall and Warren won the Nobel Prize in Medicine in 2005.[1] Medical therapy has proven to be largely successful in combating Hp.[2,3] The treatment of peptic ulcer has now changed from surgical to medical **(Figs. 1A and B)**.

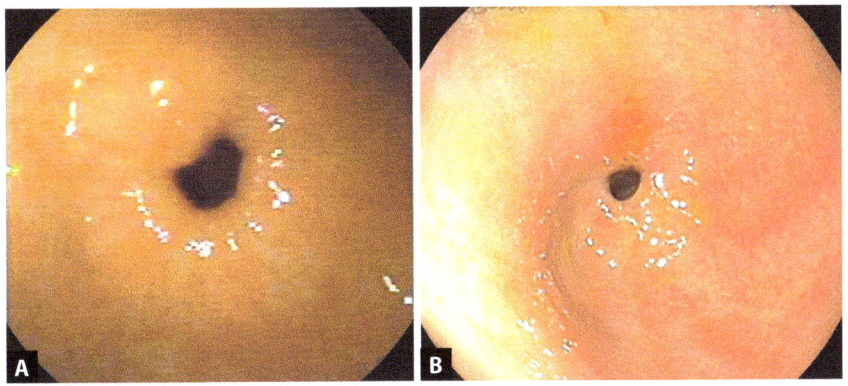

Figs. 1A and B: (A) Normal stomach in endoscopy; (B) *Helicobacter pylori* antral gastritis.

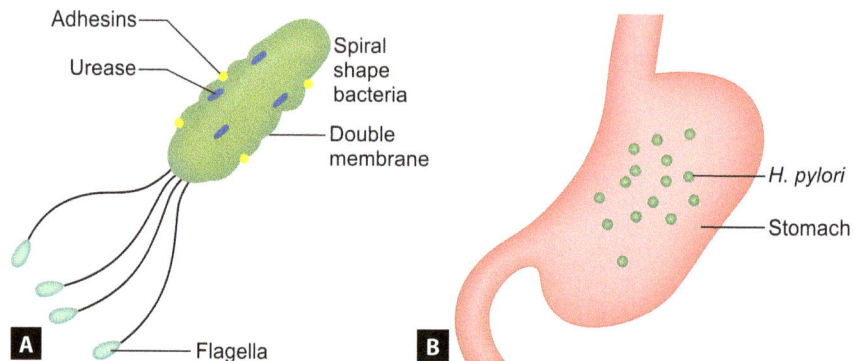

Figs. 2A and B: (A) *Helicobacter pylori* bacterium; (B) *Helicobacter pylori* bacteria in stomach.

Helicobacter pylori infection can cause gastritis, peptic ulcerations, and even gastric cancer. A persistent infection with Hp causes inflammation of gastric mucosa and gradually causes atrophy of gastric glands and low production of gastric acid. Later if not treated well, it can lead to gastric carcinoma. The World Health Organization (WHO) is of opinion that eradication of *H. pylori* is best way to prevent gastric cancer. The relationship between Hp infection and GERD is a subject of debate **(Figs. 2A and B)**.

Many epidemiological studies have shown a protective role of Hp infection toward GERD. It has been observed by various researchers that in a patient of GERD Hp infection occurs at a lower rate.

Controversy still exists about the association between GERD and Hp infection.[4]

Clinical manifestations of Hp infection include chronic gastritis, GU, and DU. Some cases of Hp infection having gastritis may not suffer with any symptoms.

It is found by various studies that if the Hp infection predominantly affects antral area of stomach then it can increase gastric acid production and can result in duodenitis and even DUs. If Hp infection affects mainly the body of stomach excluding fundus and antral parts of stomach, it can lead to low production of acid and may increase the risk of gastric carcinoma. While pangastric infection leads to gastric atrophy and increases the chances of gastric carcinoma. Antral involvement by Hp causes hyperacidity and acid reflux but after Hp eradication therapy it improves. Atrophic changes markedly increase the risk of gastric ulceration and noncardiac gastric adenocarcinomas[5,6] but the lower acid production protects against acid-induced complication of gastroesophageal reflux.[7]

McColl et al., mentions that some researchers claim that incidence of Hp infection has declined directly proportional to the decline of peptic ulcer disease[8] and an increase of reflux esophagitis but to understand current data reported on this topic it is important to distinguish between GERD symptoms, erosive esophagitis, Barrett's esophagus, and adenocarcinoma.[9]

■ REFERENCES

1. The Nobel Prize. (2005). The Nobel Prize in Physiology or Medicine 2005. [online] Available from: Nobelprize.org [Last accessed September, 2023].
2. Fennerty MB, Lieberman DA, Vakil N, Magart N, Faigel DO, Helfand M. Effectiveness of helicobacter pylori therapies in a clinical practice setting. Arch Int Med. 1999; 159(14):1562-6.

3. Rokkas T, Gisbert JP, Malfertheiner P, Niv Y, Gasbarrini A, Leja M, et al. Comparative effectiveness of multiple different first line treatment regimen for helicobacter pylori infection: a network meta-analysis. Gastroenterology. 2021;161(2):495-507.
4. Polat FR, Polat S. The effect of Helicobacter pylori or gastroesophageal reflux disease. JSLS. 2012;16(2):260-3.
5. Michael FMD, Path FRC, Genta RM, Corre Yardley J. Classification and grading of gastritis: The updated Sydney System. Am J Surg Pathol. 2010;34:434.
6. Polk DB, Peek RM. Helicobacter pylori: Gastric cancer and beyond. Nat Rev Cancer. 2010;10:403-14.
7. Mario FD, Goni E. Gastric acid secretion: changes during a century. Best Pract Res Clin Gastroenterol. 2014;28:953-65.
8. McColl KEL. Helicobactor pylori infections. N Eng J Med. 2010;362:1597-604.
9. Vasalls R, Malfurtheiner P, Kandulski A. Helicobacter pylori and non-malignant upper gastrointestinal diseases. Helicobacter 2016;21:30-33.

CHAPTER 17

Recent Advancements and Modern Trends in Gastroesophageal Reflux Disease

The main purpose of science is simplicity and as we understand more things, everything is becoming simpler.

–Edward Teller

The incidence of gastroesophageal reflux disease (GERD) is increasing world over so researchers are also struggling to find better and curative treatment for GERD. Following are the ongoing researches:
- Radiofrequency ablation (RFA)
- Transoral incisionless fundoplication (TIF)
- Medigus ultrasonic surgical endostapler (MUSE)
- Antireflux mucosectomy (ARMS)
- Bravo-Methodist Medical Center uses this small device in esophagus measuring gastric acid levels and causes of it.
- LINX-Reflux Management System (Torax Medical, Maple Grove, MN). It is a device for magnetic sphincter augmentation (MSA). It is alternative to surgical fundoplication.[1]

REFERENCE

1. LINX Management System: Safety and Effectiveness Analysis.

CHAPTER 18

Pharmacology of Drugs Used in Gastroesophageal Reflux Disease

People tend to complicate their own life, as if they were not already complicated enough.
–Carlos Ruiz Zafon

■ ANTACIDS

Antacids are drugs, which neutralize acid in stomach and relieve heartburn and indigestion. Antacids treat GERD only symptomatically that they relieve symptoms temporarily. They only neutralize the acid present in the stomach and do not reduce the acid secretion in the stomach.

■ ALGINIC ACID ANTACIDS

These are made from acid seaweed and make a film over gastric acid and thus make a barrier to acid reflux and also they neutralize the stomach acid.

H$_2$-Receptor Antagonist

H$_2$-receptor blockers or antagonists block the action of histamine on H$_2$-receptors. The hydrochloric acid is produced by parietal cells.

H$_2$-receptor antagonist are more effective in milder form of esophagitis and specially on nocturnal acid secretion. Common H$_2$-receptor antagonists are:
- Cimetidine
- Famotidine
- Ranitidine
- Nizatidine

■ SIDE EFFECTS OF H$_2$-RECEPTOR ANTAGONISTS

H$_2$-receptor antagonists are generally safe drugs as they do not cause serious side effects. Common side effects of H$_2$-receptor antagonists are:
- Headache
- Dry mouth
- Sleeping disturbances
- Dry skin
- Tinnitus
- Runny nose

■ PROTON PUMP INHIBITORS

Proton pump inhibitors (PPIs) inhibit stomach's H$^+$ K$^+$ ATPase proton pump and cause profound and prolonged reduction of gastric acid secretion.[1] PPIs are better than H$_2$-receptor antagonists.[2]

Proton pump inhibitors are used globally.[3]

Side Effects of Proton Pump Inhibitors

Numerous studies have demonstrated over prescription of PPIs.[4]

Side effects of PPIs are usually rare and are headache, nausea, diarrhea, dizziness, rash, abdominal pain, and constipation. The long-term side effects of PPIs are observed and found to be infection, fractures, kidney disease, and dementia. PPIs should not be used for long duration.[5]

PROKINETIC DRUGS

Prokinetic drugs increase gastrointestinal mobility. They increase the strength of contractions of gastrointestinal tract (GIT) muscles. They also strengthen LES. They are also called propulsive drugs as they help in forward movement of GIT contents. They are helpful in treatment of GERD. Commonly used prokinetics are:

- Domperidone
- Levosulpiride
- Itopride
- Cisapride

Common side effects of prokinetic drugs are:
- Abdominal pain
- Nausea
- Vomiting
- Diarrhea
- Depression
- Drowsiness
- Blurred vision

Certain neurosurgical problems and muscle spasms are also found in prokinetic users.

REFERENCES

1. Sachs G, Shin JM, Howdeev CW. Review article: The clinical pharmacology of proton pump inhibitors. Aliment Pharmacol Ther. 2006;23:2-8.
2. Sandhu DS, Fass R. Current trends in the management of gastroesophageal reflux disease. Gut Liver. 2018;12(1):7-16.
3. World Health Organization. World Health Organization model list of essential medicines, 21st list 2019. Geneva: World Health Organization; 2019.
4. Freedberg DE, Kim LS, Yang YX. The risks and benefits of long-term use of proton pump inhibitors: expert review and best practice advice from the American Gastroenterological Association. Gastroenterology. 2017;152:706-15.
5. Song HJ, Jiang X, Henry L, Nguyen MH, Park H. Proton pump inhibitors and risk of liver cancer and mortality in patients with chronic liver disease: a systematic review and meta-analysis. Evr J Clin Pharmacol. 2020;76:851-66.

CHAPTER 19

What Questions Patient may Ask about Gastroesophageal Reflux Disease

In life they're not going to serve you lemons, they're going to serve you lemonade; and I don't really like lemonade because I have got a really bad acid reflux.
—Felicia Day

Q.1. What should I eat, I am having gastroesophageal reflux disease (GERD)?

You can follow the following regimen:
- Drink plenty of liquids.
- Avoid aerated drinks.
- Avoid alcohol.
- Avoid large meals. Eat small and frequent meals. Smaller meals will not put pressure on lower esophageal sphincter (LES) as stomach empties fast.
- Stop smoking.
- Avoid fried and fatty foods such as pizza, burger etc.
- Avoid coffee.
- Do not eat anything 2 hours before going to bed.
- Protein-rich foods such as chicken, fish, eggs, and pulses are helpful in GERD.

Fatty foods relax LES and encourage reflux leading to heartburn.

Q.2. Is there any exercise to keep GERD in control?

Following exercises will help you:
- *Anal LES exercise:* Stand straight with your knees apart around 10 inches, tighten the anal sphincter muscles for 5 seconds and then relax for 5 seconds. Do it five times. This exercise is for any age, but very helpful in old age. It can be done by patient of any age of either sex.
- Resistance training exercises.

Q.3. How do I know that I may be suffering from GERD?

If you have heartburn more than twice a week for several weeks and inspite of medical treatment of heartburn, it keeps on coming back. You may be having GERD.

Q.4. How common is GERD?

It is one of the most common problems in gastrointestinal system.

Q.5. Is GERD dangerous to life?

GERD is not a life-threatening disease, but if it lingers on for long without proper and regular treatment, it can cause serious problems such as esophagitis, Barrett's esophagus, strictures, and adenocarcinoma of esophagus.

Q.6. How GERD is diagnosed?

GERD can be diagnosed in following ways:
- History of classical symptoms
- Acid reducing drug response test
- Esophageal pH monitoring
- Esophageal manometry

- Wireless esophageal monitoring
- Upper gastrointestinal (GI) endoscopy
- Esophageal biopsy
- Barium esophageal studies.

Q.7. What should I not do, I have GERD?

Avoid poor eating habits that may trigger reflux.

Q.8. I am suffering with GERD, can I develop cancer due to GERD?

A GERD can change the inner lining of esophagus to inner lining of stomach due to constant exposure to hydrochloric acid (HCl) which is a strong and highly corrosive acid. This change of inner lining is called Barrett's esophagus which is considered as a precancerous condition.

Q.9. Can drugs also cause heartburn?

Yes, certain medicines can also cause heartburn such as medicines for high blood pressure, pain killer medicines, sleeping pills, steroids, and some antibiotics.

Q.10. Is GERD common in India?

The prevalence of GERD in India ranges from 7.6 to 30% being <10% in most population studies and higher in cohort studies.[1]

Reflux esophagitis or GERD is very common. Approximately 60% of adult population suffer from it every year.[2]

Uncomplicated GERD should be diagnosed by symptomatology and acid suppressing drug tests.

Q.11. If I leave GERD untreated what will happen?

GERD, if untreated can cause complications, some even dangerous.
- Esophagitis—inflammation of esophagus
- Esophageal ulcers
- *Barrett's esophagus:* It is a precancerous condition.
- Esophageal structures
- Cancer of esophagus.

Q.12. What factors are under your control to avoid GERD?

Factors are under your control to avoid GERD are shown in **Figure 1**.

Q.13. Can GERD affect quality of life?

Yes. GERD affects quality of life in various aspects both physical and mental.

Q.14. Is vagus nerve yoga helpful in GERD?

Vagus nerve is a parasympathetic nerve and works against sympathetic syndromes such as "fight or flight" response.

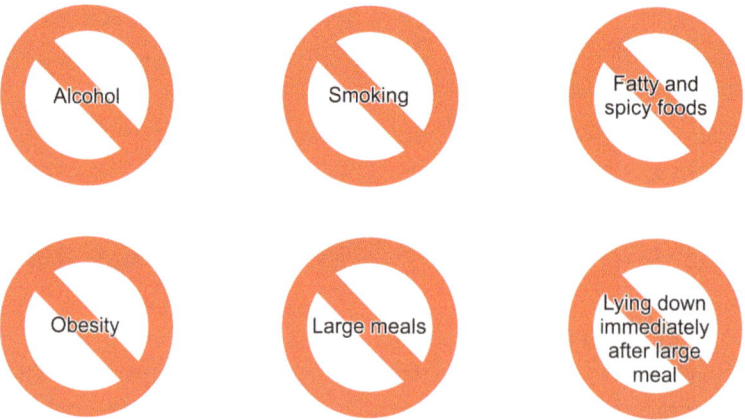

Fig. 1: Factors under your control to avoid gastroesophageal reflux disease (GERD).

Deep abdominal breathing or pranayama stimulates the vagus nerve to act opposite to fight and flight reaction. Vagus nerves stimulation creates relaxation in our body and mind. It helps in reducing the sensitivity for pain, stress, and anxiety.

Technique of Deep Abdominal Breathing[3]

When we are under stress, we breathe from the chest and it is shallow breathing. When we breathe from the diaphragm (abdominal), it is deep breathing. Shallow or chest breathing does not utilize 10–15% of lung capacity, so there is less oxygen in the blood, and also less vitality and freshness.

- Stand or sit or lie down.
- Inhale deeply from the diaphragm, pushing out the abdomen without moving your chest and count 1, 2, 3, 4 slowly in your mind while inhaling.
- Hold your breath by counting 1–16 in your mind.
- Exhale by pushing the abdomen in and not moving the chest and counting from 1 to 8 in your mind.
- Repeat it five times.

Q.15. Is heartburn a lifestyle problem?

Yes. The incidence of heartburn and GERD increases in persons with abnormal or defective lifestyle. People who are smokers or consume alcohol in large quantity or eating fried and spicy food are more prone to get heartburn **(Fig. 2)**.

Q.16. Can food cause heartburn and stimulate GERD symptoms?

Yes, some foods can precipitate GERD symptoms and some foods can relieve GERD symptoms **(Figs. 3A and B)**.

Foods to take in GERD:
- Multigrain bread

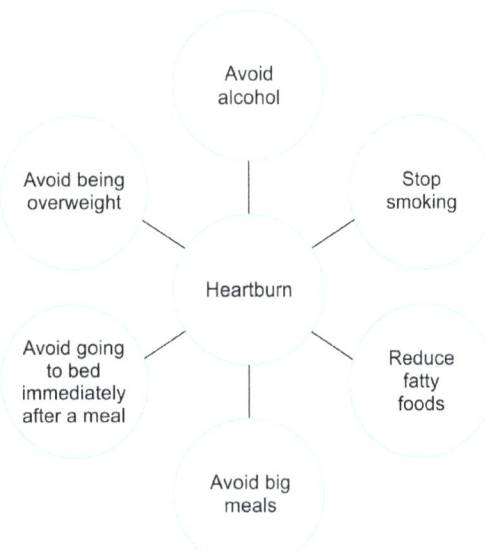

Fig. 2: Factors of heartburn.

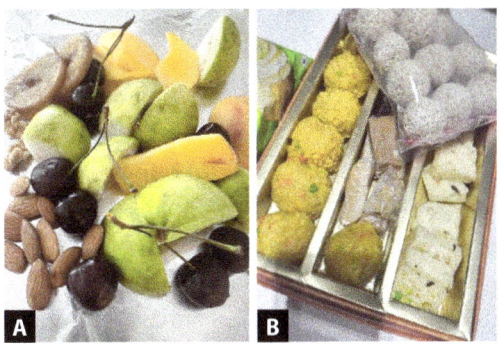

Figs. 3A and B: (A) Foods to take; (B) Foods to avoid.

- Wholegrain cereals
- Brown rice
- Noncitrus fruits
- High-protein foods
- Green leafy vegetables
- Pumpkin
- Fish, cheese, and egg white.

Foods to avoid in GERD:
- Citrus fruits
- Tomatoes
- Aerated drinks
- Coffee

- Chocolates
- Fatty and fried foods
- Spices
- Peppermint.

Q.17. Can smoking cause heartburn and how?

Smoking can cause heartburn and it does not allow ulcers to heal.
- Smoking increases production of acid by stimulating parietal cells of the stomach lining.
- Smoking relaxes LES.
- Smoking causes chemical injury to the lining of esophagus.

Q.18. Can meditation help patient of GERD?

Yes, meditation reduces stress and establishes peace and relaxation. It calms down the digestive system and makes it relaxed and rejuvenated **(Figs. 4A and B)**.

Q.19. Is there any harmful effect of hot or cold liquid and food over esophagus?

Extreme hot and cold liquids and food are not good for the health of the esophagus. Very hot beverages and food can cause thermal injuries to the walls of esophagus. There are studies which show that very hot liquids and solids may increase the risk of esophageal cancer.

Q.20. What are the most common causes of heartburn?

There are three causes which are most common in causing heartburn **(Fig. 5)**.

These are:
1. Overeating
2. Obesity and pregnancy
3. Fatty foods.

Q.21. How common is heartburn in India?

Most of the people suffer from heartburn once in a while. The prevalence of GERD in India ranges from 7.6 to 30%,[1] being <10% in most population studies, and higher in cohort studies.

Q.22. Is GERD being the other name of heartburn?

No, heartburn is a symptom and GERD is a disease. Heartburn can be caused normally also and by various other causes. A big meal can cause GERD which may cause heartburn.

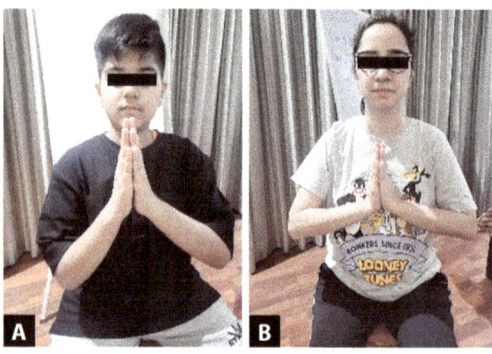

Figs. 4A and B: Meditation reduces stress.

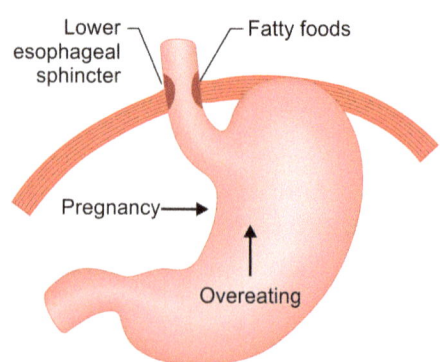

Fig. 5: Common causes of heartburn.

Q.23. What are the risk factors of GERD?

Following factors are risk factor for development of GERD:
- Obesity
- Pregnancy
- Overeating
- Hiatus hernia.

Q.24. When should you consult a doctor for GERD?

Difficulty in swallowing, painful swallowing, weight loss without attempting to reduce weight, persistent vomiting, chest pain, blood in vomit, or dark stools.

Q.25. What happens in acid reflux?

Food is carried forward in food pipe (esophagus) by peristalsis to the stomach. LES is the sphincter present at lower end of esophagus which opens and allows food to enter the stomach. Sometimes, the LES relaxes without food and allows acid of stomach to leak in esophagus leading to heartburn. This happens occasionally to every person. This usually occurs after food and at night.

When reflux occurs recurrently and is associated with symptoms it is called GERD.

Q.26. What lifestyle changes you can make in GERD to ease symptoms?

Stop smoking, reduce alcohol intake, keep ideal weight for your age and height, avoid trigger foods, do not go to bed for 3 hours after a meal, avoid heavy meal, and raise head end of your bed 6–8 inches.

Q.27. How will you doubt that you have hiatus hernia?

Usually following symptoms indicate pressure of hiatus hernia.
- Heartburn
- Nausea
- Vomiting
- Burping
- Acid regurgitation.

Q.28. Which lifestyle measure help in hiatus hernia?

Following lifestyle changes help a patient of hiatus hernia:
- Lose weight.
- Do not eat big meal instead have small meals frequently.
- Elevate head end of bed 6–8 inches.
- Do not go to bed for 3 hours after a meal.
- Reduce alcohol.
- Stop smoking.

Q.29. Can exercise help in hiatus hernia?

Following exercise help in hiatus hernia:
- Yoga
- Walking
- Jogging
- Swimming
- Meditation.

Q.30. Can hiatus hernia increase symptoms of GERD?

Yes, hiatus hernia can aggravate acid-related symptoms in GERD.

Q.31. How is hiatus hernia diagnosed?

Upper GI endoscopy.

Q.32. Can pranayama and deep abdominal breathing help in GERD?

Yes, deep abdominal breathing strengthens diaphragmatic muscles without strain.

Q.33. What exercises to be avoided by hiatus hernia patient?

Weightlifting.

Q.34. How common is hiatus hernia?

It is quite common. As our age increases the incidence of hiatus hernia increases.

Q.35. What foods to be avoided by a hiatus hernia patient?

Fatty, fried, and spicy foods to be avoided as they increase the symptoms of hiatus hernia.

Q.36. What are types or grades of GERD?

Types of GERD:
- *Stage 1:* Mild GERD—symptoms occur once or twice a month
- *Stage 2:* Moderate GERD—more frequent symptoms. Use medicines, proton pump inhibitors (PPIs), etc.
- *Stage 3:* Sever GERD—daily frequent symptoms and symptoms are not well controlled.
- *Stage 4:* Precancer GERD—long-standing GERD can cause precancerous condition.

Q.37. Is there any relation between stress and GERD?

Yes, stress can precipitate symptom of GERD. Stress increases gastric acid production and LES also works abnormally.

Q.38. Can drinking milk help in GERD?

It is a myth as milk, specially full cream is a common trigger drink. In fact, all dairy products act as trigger foods some mild and others strong.

REFERENCES

1. Bhatia SJ, Makharia GK, Abraham P, Bhat N, Reddy DN, Ghoshal UC, et al. Indian consensus on gastroesophageal reflux disease in adults: a position statement of the Indian Society of Gastroenterology. Indian J Gastroentrol. 2019;38(5):411-40.
2. Samiran N. Understanding Heartburn and Reflux Osteophagitis. India: Elsevier India; 2016.
3. Nigam VK, Nigam S. 40 Minutes with God. New Delhi: Viva Books; 2010. pp. 40.

CHAPTER 20

Some Interesting Cases of Gastroesophageal Reflux Disease

(Name of the patients changed to protect their identity)

*You cannot transmit wisdom and insight to another person. The seed is already there.
A good teacher touches the seed, allowing it to wake up, to sprout, and to grow.*
—Thich Nhat Hanh

GASTROESOPHAGEAL REFLUX DISEASE AND *HELICOBACTER PYLORI* INFECTION MADE A PATIENT'S LIFE MISERABLE BUT FOUND RELIEF WITH PROPER DIAGNOSIS AND MEDICATIONS

Mr Ahmed Hussain, a 45-year-old man, was suffering from upper abdomen and chest discomfort with nausea and occasional vomiting. He was also a heavy smoker. He was diagnosed as suffering with gastroesophageal reflux disease (GERD) and advised upper gastrointestinal endoscopy. His wife was accompanying him for the procedure. She told me that he had suddenly developed a feeling of claustrophobia whenever he was in small room or even a dark room. He will not agree for endoscopy as he is scared of a tube going down his throat and he has already refused. I trained him with technique of visualization for a few days. He felt better and agreed for endoscopy. I gave him a sedative. Upper gastrointestinal endoscopy was done successfully and we confirmed GERD and a duodenal ulcer and treated him accordingly. This is the help we can get with relaxation techniques which help to avoid anesthesia in such cases **(Figs. 1 and 2)**.

The understanding of the role of bacteria in stomach ulcers was researched in the 1970s. The bacterium had also been observed in 1979 by Australian pathologist Robin Warren, who did further research on it with Australian physician Barry Marshall beginning in 1981. After numerous unsuccessful attempts at culturing the bacteria from the stomach, they finally succeeded in visualizing the colonies in 1982, when they unintentionally left their petridishes incubating for 5 days over the Easter weekend. In their original

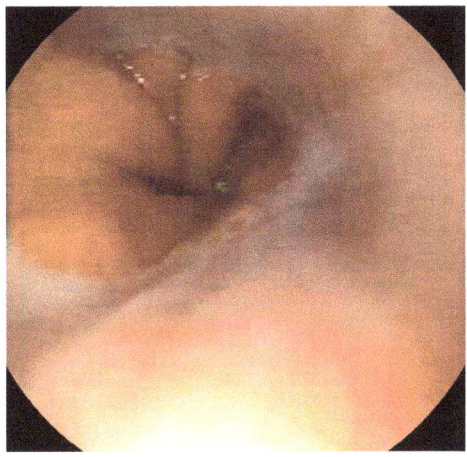

Fig. 1: Gastroesophageal reflux disease (GERD) on endoscopy.

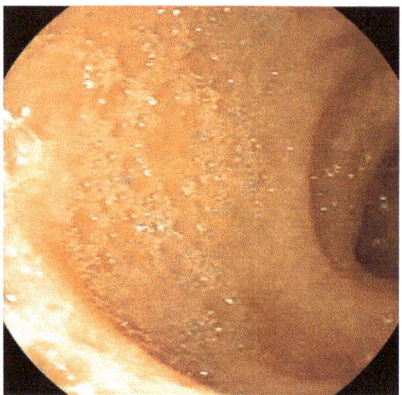

Fig. 2: Healed duodenal ulcer.

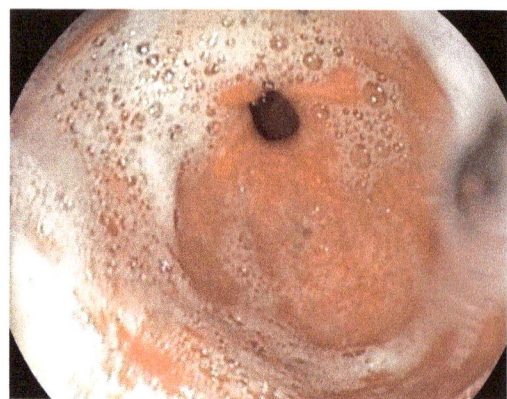

Fig. 3: Erosive antral gastritis due to *H. pylori* infection.

paper, Warren and Marshall contended that most stomach ulcers and gastritis were caused by bacteria. Marshall and Warren studied the presence of spiral bacteria in association with gastritis. The following year in 1982 they performed the initial culture of *Helicobacter pylori* (*H. pylori*) and developed their hypothesis related to the bacterial cause of peptic ulcer and gastric cancer. The *H. pylori* theory was ridiculed by scientists and doctors, who did not believe that any bacteria could live in the acidic medium of the stomach. After failed attempts to infect piglets in 1984, Marshall drank a petridish of the bacteria and soon developed gastritis with achlorhydria. Barry Marshall and Robin Warren were awarded the Nobel Prize in Physiology or Medicine in 2005. Barry Marshall rightly wrote that, "The greatest obstacle to discovery is not ignorance, it is the illusion of knowledge".

The common routes of transmission of *H. pylori* bacteria are fecal-oral and oral-oral. Contaminated water is one of the main sources of *H. pylori* bacteria. Contaminated water drinking leads to *H. pylori* gastritis, antral, or pangastritis. Some researchers have isolated and cultured *H. pylori* bacteria from drinking water indicating the source of *H. pylori*. The selection of drinking water specially by careful monitoring can reduce the risk of getting *H. pylori* infection and its complications. In keeping with this, there are some reports regarding the contamination of these kinds of water with dangerous pathogens such as *H. pylori, Vibrio cholera, Salmonella typhimurium,* and *Escherichia coli*.[1-3]

In India, especially in villages drinking of well water is very common and without knowing whether the well water is contaminated or not. Many sicknesses in Indian villagers may be contributed by the contaminated well water. In summary, the use of drinking of *H. pylori* contaminated well water appears associated with the acquisition of an *H. pylori* infection (**Figs. 3 to 5**).[4]

Helicobacter pylori are curved, gram-negative, microaerophilic bacteria[5] found in the gastric mucous layer or adherent to the epithelial lining of the stomach.[6] It has been a public health significance bacteria since 1983 as it infects the duodenum where hydrochloric acid and pepsin play a role in the digestion of food, which facilitates damage of the lining by gastric acid.[7] *H. pylori* can elevate acid secretion in people who develop duodenal ulcers[8] or hypersecretion of gastric acid can by itself evoke duodenal ulcers.[9]

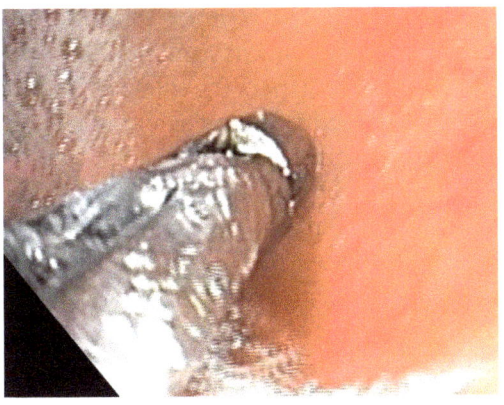

Fig. 4: Endoscopic biopsy from antral gastritis area.

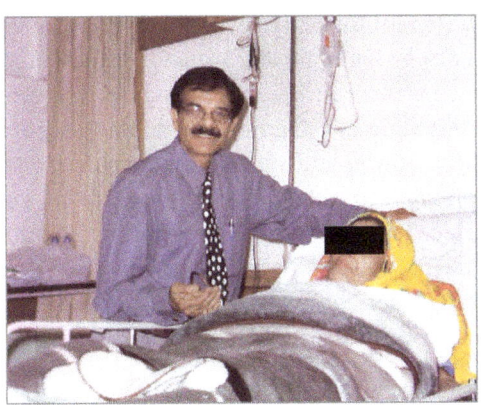

Fig. 6: Author with the patient.

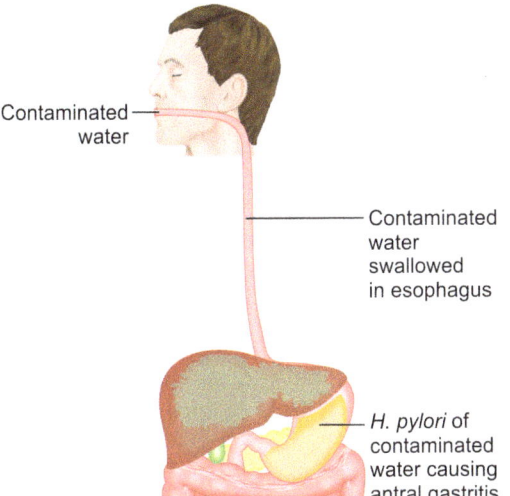

Fig. 5: Contaminated water leads to gastritis, antral, or pan gastritis.

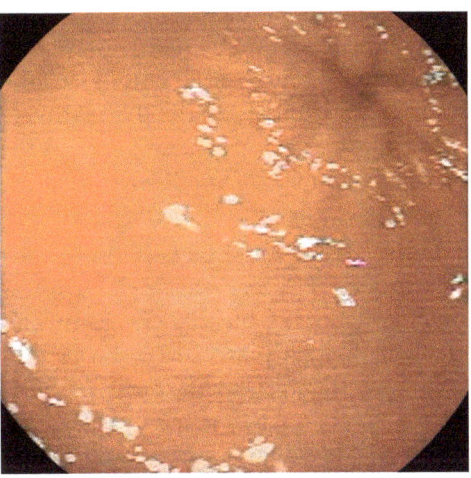

Fig. 7: Prepyloric gastritis on endoscopy.

A BLIND GIRL SUFFERING DUE TO GASTROESOPHAGEAL REFLUX DISEASE AND *H. PYLORI* GASTRITIS

I was working as Chief Surgeon and Director of Aden Refinery Company Hospital, Aden, Yemen from 1983 to 2000. In Aden, GERD and *H. pylori* gastritis were very common. It was probably due to chewing of a herb *"Qat"*, which gives a mild intoxicating effect. Most of adults used to chew *"Qat"* on every weekend. Some people were so addicted that they used to chew daily. There was a 30-year-old female named Fatima, who was my patient, in the early '80s. She was suffering with severe gastritis and duodenal ulcer. Unfortunately, Fatima was blind. I used to perform operations for duodenal ulcers, but unfortunately the recurrence rate was quite high, operation was not a cure. Fatima refused for surgery and requested for conservative treatment **(Figs. 6 and 7)**.

Fatima used to come to my OPD with severe pain. After sitting on the patient's chair, she used to remove her veil and gloves and used to cry saying, "Doctor either kill me or cure me. I cannot tolerate this pain of abdomen. It is very severe". I used to pacify her by giving some medicine for pain as there was no ulcer healing medicines at that time and telling her, "Fatima, try this medicine it will help you and should not eat spicy food". Fatima used to tell, "Sir, I am not taking any spicy food, I am only on bread and cold milk. Cold milk gives me some relief, but again pain starts after some time". She used to depart with a heavy heart and depressed.

I remember that when ulcer healing medicine, tagamet (cimetidine) was introduced for the first time for gastritis, ulcers, and GERD **(Fig. 8)**, it was very costly medicine at that time and not easily available. I prescribed a course of tagamet for Fatima and when she came I prescribed and arranged for her. She was still depressed and told me that, "I have lost faith in medicines, but as you are advising I will take this medicine also".

I was very happy when I saw Fatima next week in my OPD. She was smiling, for the first time, and she blessed me from heart for alleviating her pain. She departed with, "Thank you Doctor, God bless you".

H. pylori is a gram-negative microaerophilic bacterium, that generally colonizes the stomach in early life.[10] It has the ability to reach the protective mucous layer at the surface of gastric mucosa and to survive the extreme acid content of the stomach. Thanks to its 4–6 flagella, and by avoiding low pH areas using chemotaxis it first colonizes the antrum, where there are no acid-producer cells.[11,12] It produces a huge amount of urease, that metabolizes the urea present in the stomach in ammonia and carbon dioxide in order to produce a neutralized area where the bacteria can live.[13]

CHILD SUFFERING FROM GASTROESOPHAGEAL REFLUX DISEASE

Master Dhruv, a premature child, who is now 11 years old, was having repeated vomiting especially when he was having a heavy meal with tomatoes and chocolates. Parents were very worried as it was affecting his studies and health **(Figs. 9 and 10)**.

Everybody of his family was advising him about overeating at the time of lunch and dinner. He was also psychologically disturbed. Many physicians and pediatricians were consulted and everybody felt it was overeating and prescribed antacids. He was not cured. He continued suffering till the parents met

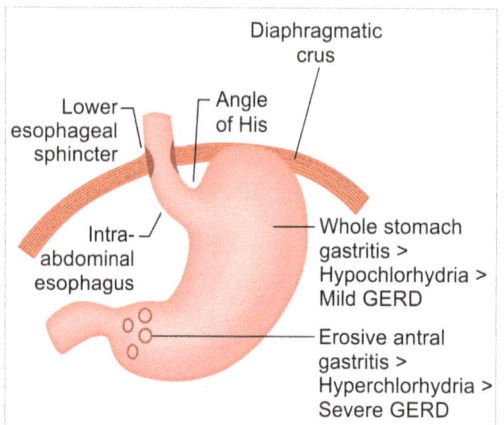

Fig. 8: Gastroesophageal reflux disease (GERD) due to antral and pangastritis.

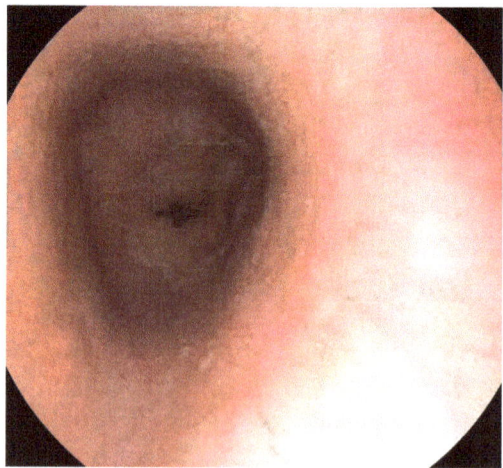

Fig. 9: Normal esophagus on endoscopy.

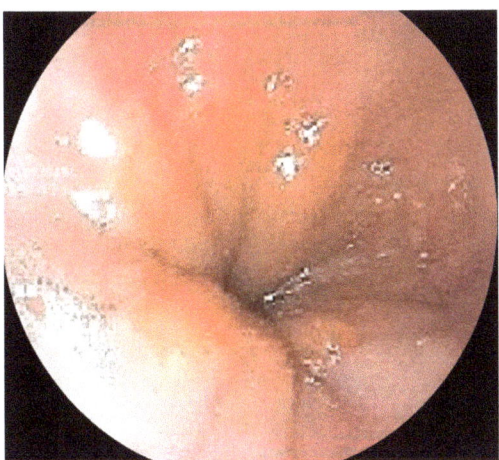

Fig. 10: Gastroesophageal reflux disease (GERD) on endoscopy.

Gastroesophageal reflux disease is common in premature children. Gastroesophageal reflux (GER) is common in newborn babies and more so in premature babies. The normal or physiological GER usually resolves at the birth or by first birthday (1 year). GERD is common in overweight children so if the premature child is overweight, he has all the chances of developing GERD. Many infants in the neonatal intensive care unit (NICU) are prescribed acid suppressive therapies to treat a presumed diagnosis of GERD.[14,15]

PATIENT ALMOST LOST HIS VOICE DUE TO GASTROESOPHAGEAL REFLUX DISEASE

an experienced gastroenterologist who diagnosed it as GERD. He explained that it is common in premature children. He did upper gastrointestinal endoscopy and GERD was diagnosed. The gastroesophageal junction was patulous and lower esophageal sphincter (LES) was relaxed. He advised the following treatment and lifestyle guidelines:

- Take food in small quantity and frequently and avoid a big meal.
- Avoid chocolates and foods with chocolate in them.
- Avoid tomatoes.
- Change the diet, to add plenty of fruits and vegetables.
- Reduce fatty and fried foods.
- Reduce aerated drinks and coffee.
- Sleep, 2 hours after dinner and better to walk after lunch and dinner for 10 minutes.
- While sleeping, raise headend by two pillows.
- Advised to take proton pump inhibitors (PPIs) and antacid gel for 8 weeks.

He took medicines for 8 weeks and improved a lot, but he still continues to follow lifestyle changes advised to him. He is now in class 6 and is doing very well with study and sports.

Heartburn and indigestion are common problems that people neglect and use home remedies without knowing that it may lead to serious sickness if neglected. Mr Mathur was suffering from burning in throat, chest, and upper abdomen. He used to take cold milk and cold water to tackle this problem. He never consulted a doctor, gradually he felt that his voice was becoming hoarse and weak, so he consulted a doctor who after hearing his story and examination referred him to a gastroenterologist who did upper gastrointestinal endoscopy and diagnosed him as suffering with GERD **(Figs. 11 and 12)**.

He was also advised to change his diet, raise the head end of the bed, and go to bed at least 2 hours after meals. He prescribed him to take PPI in two divided doses along with antacids. He started feeling better and continued PPI for 4 weeks in two divided doses, then was advised to take PPI for only once a day for 4 weeks and then gradually diminish the dose and stop. He is fine now and managing with only lifestyle changes.

The term "laryngopharyangeal reflux disease (reflux laryngitis)" was adopted in 2002 by the American Academy of

Otolaryangology and Head and Neck Surgery and reference to clinical manifestations of gastric reflux on the upper airways.[16-18] This supraesophageal form of GERD was named in 1994 by Koufman and Cummins,[19] not with the intention to designate the original reflux, but to call attention to the predominance of symptoms and changes in the laryngopharyngeal segment.[20] Usually, the reflux laryngitis due to GERD makes the voice hoarse, but sometimes it can completely make the voice disappear as happened in our case.

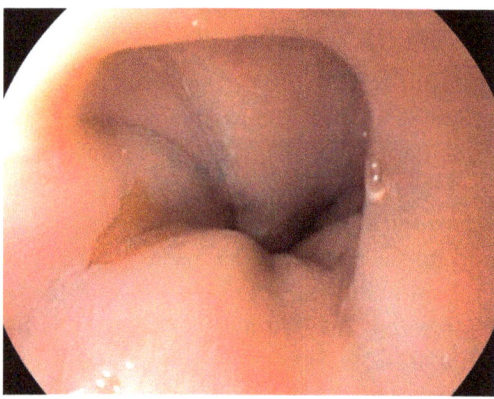

Fig. 11: Gastroesophageal reflux disease (GERD) on endoscopy.

PATIENT WITH HIATUS HERNIA AND GASTROESOPHAGEAL REFLUX DISEASE

Mrs Shanti Jain, aged 42 years old, was suffering with heartburn, pain, and discomfort in lower chest and upper abdomen, bloating, burping, bitter taste, sour eructations, nausea, and sometimes vomiting. She occasionally used to feel like food was getting stuck in chest. She was using home remedies and antacids and getting relief, but when food started getting stuck in the chest, she consulted a gastroenterologist. He did upper gastrointestinal endoscopy and diagnosed as suffering with GERD and small hiatus hernia. She was advised some lifestyle changes, antacids, PPI, and a prokinetic drug **(Figs. 13 to 16)**. She was advised following lifestyle changes:

- Recognize trigger foods and avoid them.
- Eat small meals frequently and avoid a big meal.
- Avoid fatty and fried foods, alcohol, chocolate, tomatoes, aerated drinks, and coffee.
- Not to lie down immediately after meals.
- Raise head end of bed by 6-9 inch or use two pillows while on bed.
- Do regular exercise to keep weight in normal range.

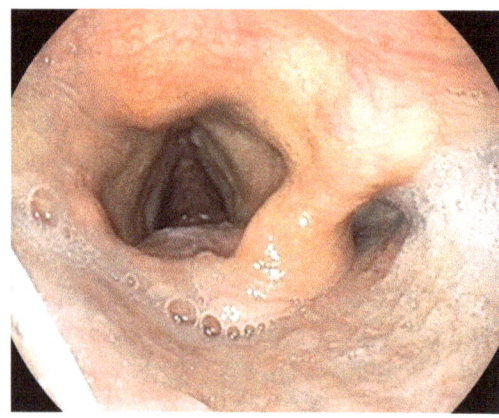

Fig. 12: Laryngitis due to gastroesophageal reflux disease (GERD).

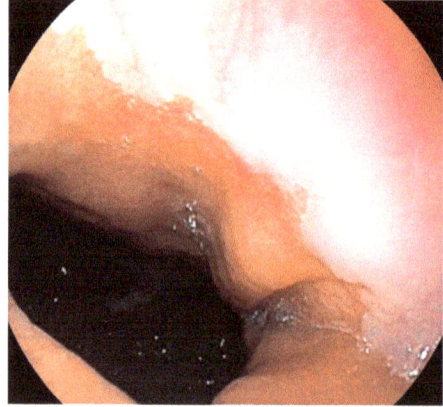

Fig. 13: Hiatus hernia with gastroesophageal reflux disease (GERD)

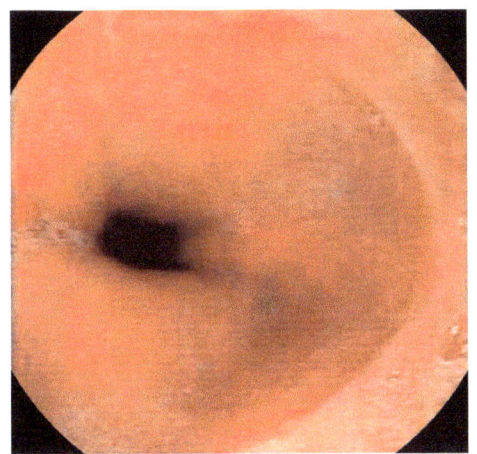

Fig. 14: Eight weeks after treatment.

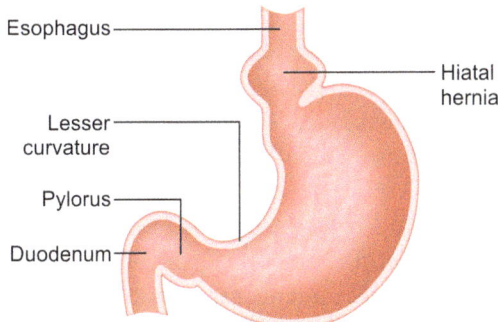

Fig. 15: Hiatal hernia.

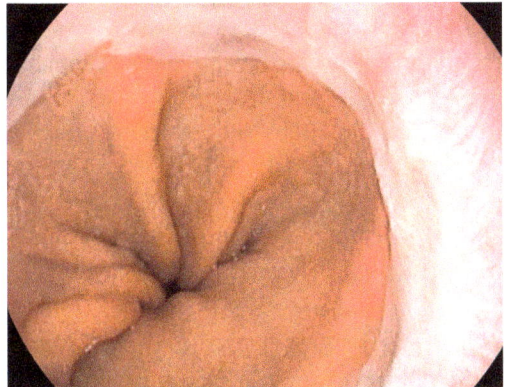

Fig. 16: Hiatus hernia with gastroesophageal reflux disease (GERD) on endoscopy.

No surgery was advised for hiatus hernia. She improved with her lifestyle changes.

Historically, hypotheses on the pathogeneses of GERD have been implicated either anatomical or physiological abnormalities of the gastroesophageal junction.[21] Recent evidence suggests that dominant mechanism may vary as a function of disease severity with transient LES relaxation predominating with mild disease and mechanisms associated with a hiatus hernia and/or weak sphincter dominating with more severe disease.[22] Patients with hiatus hernia exhibit progressive disruption of the diaphragmatic sphincter proportional to the extent of axial herniation. Therefore, although neither condition in and of itself (hiatus hernia or hypotensive LES) results in severe incompetence, the two conditions interact with each other as evidenced by the statistical modeling of gastroesophageal junction competence......[23]

Hiatus hernia (HH) interferes with the anatomy and physiology of the normal antireflux barrier through several mechanisms, ...[24] Hiatus hernia is a known risk factor for GERD since it impairs the esophagogastric junction, leading to reduction in lower sphincter junction pressure; increase in the frequency of the transient lower esophageal sphincter relaxation; and impairment of esophageal clearance.[25]

PATIENT WITH GASTROESOPHAGEAL REFLUX DISEASE WITH BARRETT'S ESOPHAGUS

Mr Jai Prakash Srivastava, a 49-year-old male businessman, was suffering with heartburn and occasional mild pain in upper abdomen. One day while in a meeting, he developed sudden severe pain in lower chest and upper abdomen. The pain was so severe that he felt as he had heart attack. He was taken to a nearby hospital where he got admitted in intensive care unit (ICU). Electrocardiogram

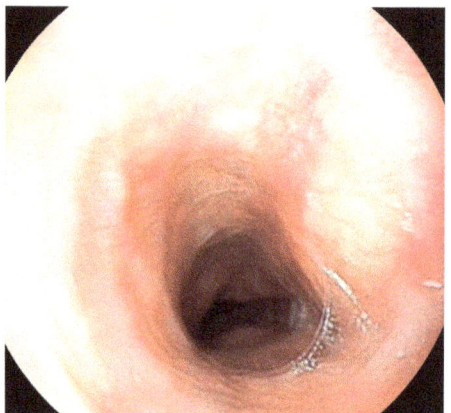

Fig. 17: Barrett's esophagus.

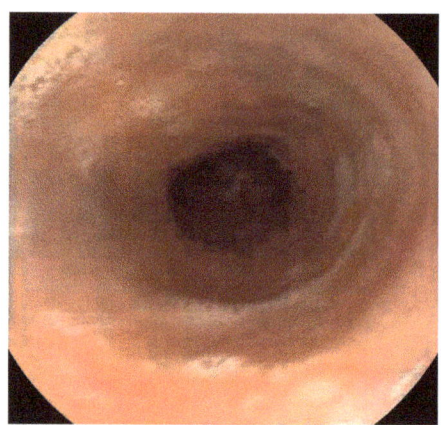

Fig. 18: 3 months after treatment.

(ECG) and other tests for heart attack were normal and so cardiac cause was ruled out. A gastroenterologist was called who took thorough history and examined him, then did upper gastrointestinal endoscopy. He diagnosed him as suffering with GERD with Barrett's esophagus (BE). Barrett's esophagus was confirmed by biopsy. Barrett's esophagus is a premalignant condition. Barrett's esophagus occurs in people who suffer from GERD as the refluxed acid burns the lining of the lower esophagus **(Figs. 17 and 18)**.

He was advised lifestyle changes and medications. He was advised to get regular follow-ups especially endoscopy and biopsy. His follow-up endoscopies showed improvement and he also felt better symptomatically.

Gastroesophageal reflux disease is an important disease as its complications can be serious and can prove fatal. GERD, if neglected and untreated for long, can develop Barrett's esophagus which is a precancerous condition **(Figs. 19A to D)**. GERD is considered as primary risk factor for Barrett's esophagus. The acid refluxate in esophagus from stomach leads to the injury to the lining of lower esophagus which predisposes it for Barrett's esophagus. The relationships among GERD, Barrett's esophagus, and esophageal adenocarcinoma are clearly established. Duration and severity of GERD symptoms increase risk not only for Barrett's esophagus, but also for esophageal adenocarcinoma; in fact, patients with severe and prolonged symptoms of GERD have an odd ratio of 43.5 for development of esophageal adenocarcinoma compared with patient who did not report any recurrent GERD symptoms.[26,27]

GERD, Barrett's esophagus, and esophageal adenocarcinoma have all been associated with the presence of obesity. The relationship between GERD and obesity is thought to be in part due to increased gastroesophageal sphincter gradient (Mercer et al., 1987),[28] intra-abdominal pressure (El-Serag et al., 2006b),[29] an increased incidence of hiatal hernia in obesity (Pandolfino et al., 2006).[30]

SHE SUFFERED WITH GASTROESOPHAGEAL REFLUX DISEASE, HIATUS HERNIA, AND UMBILICAL HERNIA

Mrs Shreedevi, a 40-year-old lady, was a school teacher of class 8th, 9th, and 10th. She

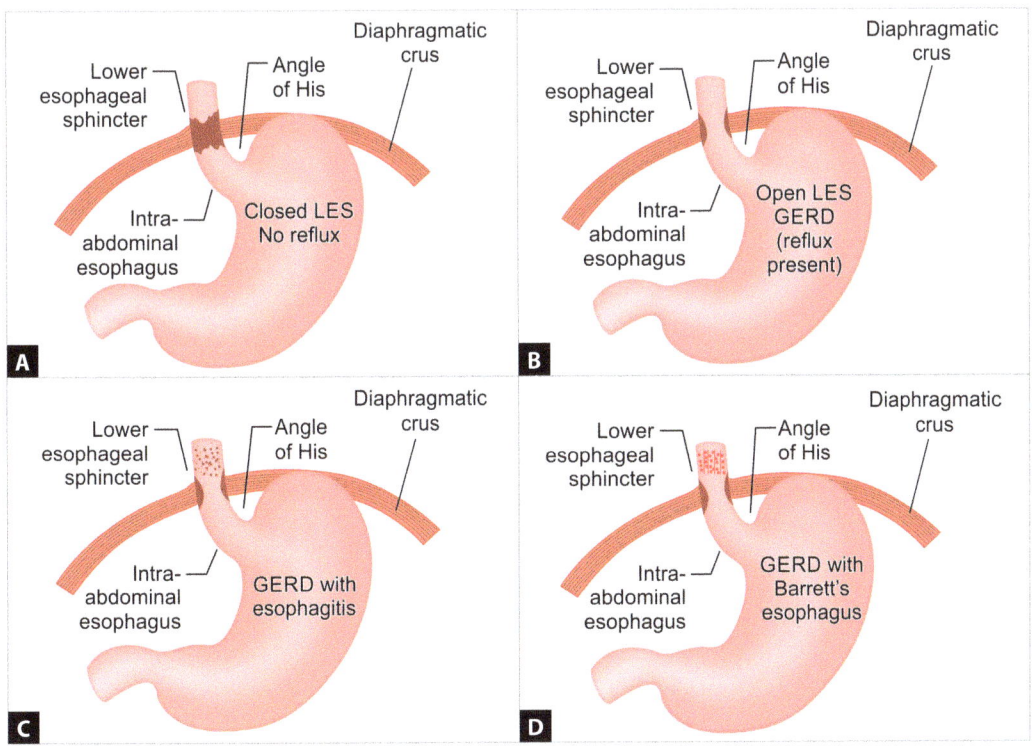

Figs. 19A to D: Neglected and untreated gastroesophageal reflux disease (GERD) can lead to Barrett's esophagus.

used to teach children chemistry. She was a jolly, happy, and talkative person, probably due to her subject. She used to take interest in teaching and devoting time to prepare for her classes. She loved her work and was usually up early and out of the home by 1 hour before time so that to reach in time to school as there may be traffic on the way. She often devoted whole evening planning for lessons for next day. Over time she noticed that after breakfast or small meal her tummy became distended and tense with burning sensations in upper part of abdomen. Often she felt nauseated and occasionally vomited. She took ENO fruit salt and sometimes cold milk and digene syrup. She continued with these measures but later on she started having pain in lower part of chest with burning sensation. Same time her stress increased as layoffs started at her school. Now she was too much disturbed due to her sickness and fear of losing her job. This stress increased the severity of her symptoms of pain in chest and burning sensations. She visited a private doctor. He advised her to take syrup of algenic acid, a prokinetic, and take small frequent meals rather big meals. She continued the treatment and small meals but nothing happened so she visited a big private hospital when she was seen by a specialist who advised her few tests and upper gastrointestinal endoscopy. At last, she was diagnosed having GERD, hiatus hernia, and a big umbilical hernia. She was given treatment for GERD, PPI, and prokinetic for 4 weeks with some lifestyle changes. She was also advised to go for operation for her big umbilical hernia. She felt better and got her

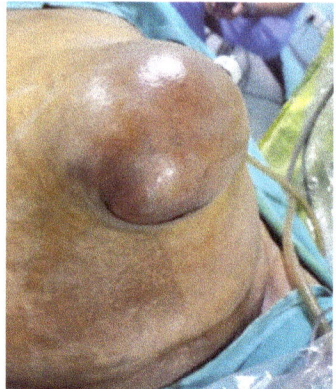

Fig. 20: Huge umbilical hernia.

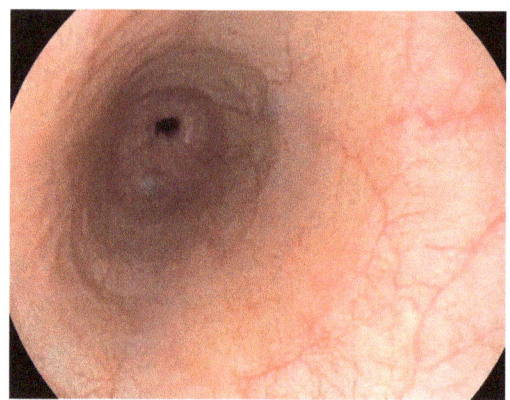

Fig. 22: Open lower esophageal sphincter (LES).

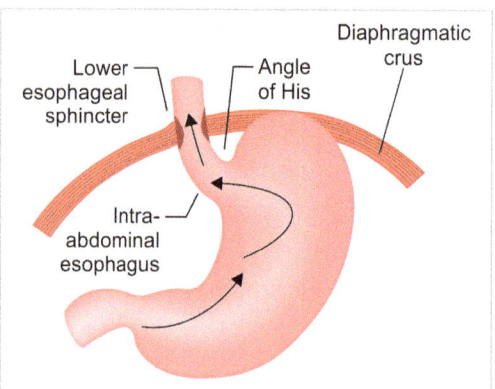

Fig. 21: Acid and gastric content reflux from stomach to esophagus in huge umbilical hernia due to traction on herniated loops of bowel.

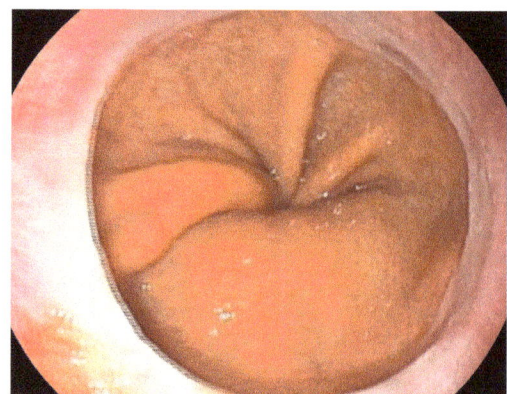

Fig. 23: Gastroesophageal reflux disease (GERD) with hiatus hernia.

umbilical hernia operated and continued her medicines for further 4 weeks as advised by specialist doctor. Today she is almost got cured of her ailments **(Figs. 20 and 21)**.

It is not uncommon to find a patient suffering with GERD and hiatus hernia also suffering with abdominal wall hernia. The pathogenesis of hiatus hernia and abdominal wall hernias is similar as in both high intra-abdominal pressure is one of the main causative factors. Though these two hernias are different entities but are seen together sometimes. Similarly, one of the risk factors for GERD is increased intra-abdominal pressure leading to weak LES causing reflux of gastric contents to esophagus. It can be either way as a person suffering with abdominal wall hernia can develop GERD or a person suffering with GERD can develop abdominal wall hernia. A retrospective study found that the incidence of inguinal hernia was 2.5 times higher in patients with history of hiatus hernia **(Figs. 22 and 23)**.[31]

Meta-analysis of 25,310 patients found that obesity doubled the risk of hiatus hernia.[32] Obesity has also been identified as a risk factor for abdominal wall hernias in both retrospective and prospective studies.[33,34]

SHE SUFFERED WITH BOTH GASTROESOPHAGEAL REFLUX DISEASE AND CHRONIC CHOLELITHIASIS (GALLSTONES)

Mrs Kusum Yadav, aged 35 years, was a brilliant executive in her public relation field. She earned this name by working hard with devotion without thinking about time she gave to her profession and organization. One night while sleeping, she suddenly felt severe pain in upper abdomen. The pain was so severe that she could not sit and was bending forward. She vomited also once. With great difficulty she rang her mother in downstairs and called her. Seeing her suffering, family members took her to a nearby hospital. She was seen by the doctor on duty and was advised for admission. In the casualty department, she was given intravenous drip, and intravenous pain killer which helped her by reducing the pain. During this time, she also developed mild fever and shivering. She also gave history of heartburn and upper abdominal discomfort and mild dull pain off and on for the last 2 years. She noticed that heartburn and abdominal discomfort used to increase whenever she was under stress but she never had such severe pain in abdomen and vomiting. She used to get relief by cold milk and bland diet. Some tests, ultrasound of abdomen and upper gastrointestinal endoscopy revealed that she was suffering with GERD and cholelithiasis (gallstones) **(Fig. 24)**. There were multiple stones in the gall bladder from 2 to 12 mm. Next day, she was posted for laparoscopic cholecystectomy and was discharged after the day of operation with advice to eat small meals four to five times instead two big meals and walk for 10–15 minutes after each meal and wait for at least 2 hours to go to bed after a meal. Avoid aerated drinks, alcohol, and fatty and spicy foods. She was advised PPI in two doses daily for 8 weeks and a prokinetic for 4 weeks.

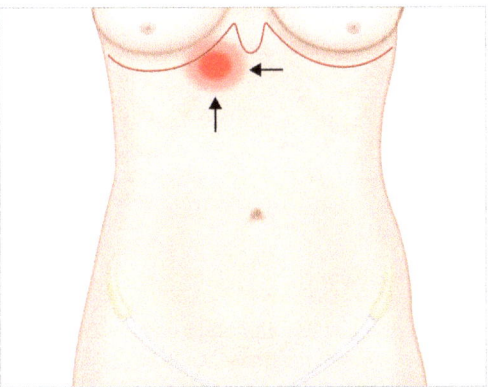

Fig. 24: Site of pain and tenderness in gallstones.

Now she is a relieved healthy woman without any heartburn or pain.

Gastroesophageal reflux disease and cholelithiasis (gallstones) are separate entities. Both ailments are related with different organs. GERD with esophagus and stomach while cholelithiasis with gallbladder. They are different diseases but their symptoms may be similar. Heartburn and abdominal pain associated with fatty food are frequently noticed in both the GERD and gallstone disease. Being overweight, lying down after eating and frequently eating fatty and spicy foods make confusion regarding the diagnosis of ailment. If the abdominal pain, heartburn, and indigestion are associated with fever and shivering, one must report to the doctor.

Some researchers feel that there is a link between cholelithiasis and cholecystectomy and GERD, but there is no proper evidence of association between these were found. In Brazil, evaluating 3,934 individuals, Oliveira SS et al.[35] obtained prevalence of 31.3% for GERD, more common in women. The association between cholelithiasis and GERD remains uncertain. In two studies, the relationship between them was not found, Avidan B et al.[36] evaluated

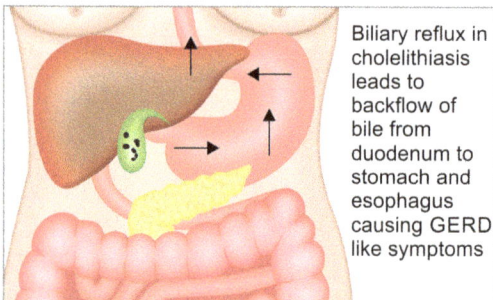

Fig. 25: Biliary reflux leading to gastroesophageal reflux disease (GERD).

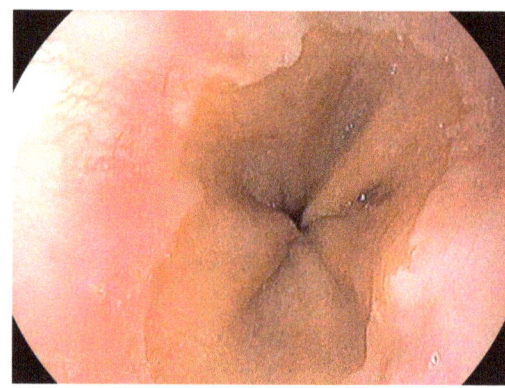

Fig. 27: Gastroesophageal reflux disease (GERD) on endoscopy.

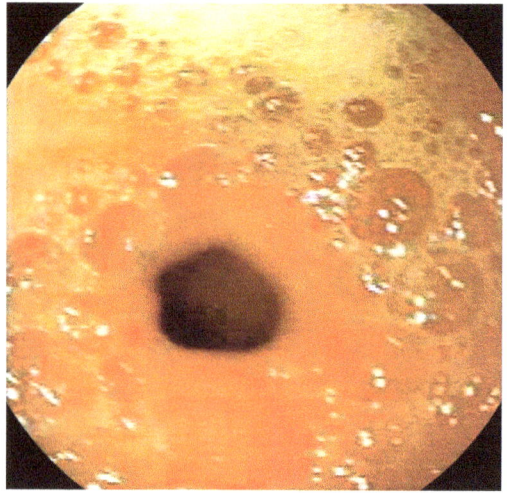

Fig. 26: Biliary reflux.

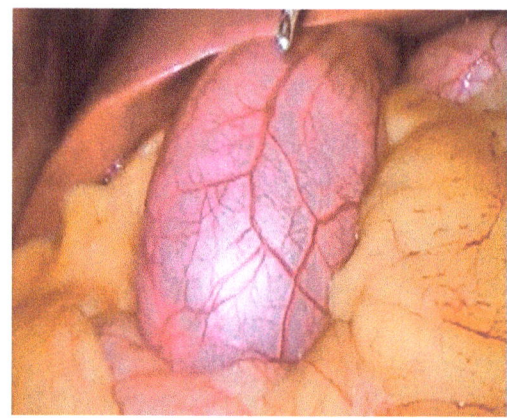

Fig. 28: Gallbladder with stones during laparoscopic cholecystectomy.

on a case-control study, while Martinez Pancarbo C et al.[37] a transversal cohort study. Nowadays, especially with the advent of video laparoscopic treatment of esophageal diseases, the diagnosis of cholelithiasis is especially important due to the possibility of simultaneous surgical treatment of esophageal and biliary disorders in a minimally invasive procedures **(Figs. 25 and 26)**.[38]

It is so far not proved that there is link between gallstone disease and GERD, but bile reflux from duodenum to stomach and sometimes to esophagus specially if the LES is weak and incompetent can cause GERD like symptoms. Bile reflux is quite common in gallstone disease leading to gallbladder dyspepsia **(Figs. 27 and 28)**.

HE WAS A SMOKER AND SUFFERING WITH COMORBIDITIES (OBESITY AND HYPERTENSION) AND THEN DEVELOPED GASTROESOPHAGEAL REFLUX DISEASE

Mr Srikant, a 50-year-old male, had a decent job with normal health, but gradually he found loss of energy with development of extreme weakness. He used to get breathless while walking fast or going up with stairs. This increased his anxiety. As this was not enough, his wife suddenly died which stimulated a severe bout of depression which increased his sufferings. He consulted an internal medicine consultant who after investigating him for his breathlessness, upper abdominal discomfort, heartburn, and occasional severe headaches. He diagnosed him as suffering with uncontrolled hypertension, obesity, and GERD. Doctor found after discussion with Mr Srikant that he was not taking care of his health though he was depressed due to the demise of his wife. Specialist encouraged him to take care of his health so as to look after his children. Ultimately, he agreed and started regular mild exercises and medicines. He also underwent abdominal ultrasound and upper gastrointestinal tract endoscopy. Gradually, his symptoms of GERD subsided with lifestyle changes and treatment. He found that PPI which was prescribed by the doctor helped him a lot. His blood pressure also got reduced and came within normal range according to his age. His weight did not reduce but also did not increase, remained stationary, but he found himself more alert and energetic **(Figs. 29 and 30)**.

Obesity is diagnosed when the body mass index (BMI) is 30 kg/m² or more. Earlier obesity was a prevalent feature in western world, but now it is increasing in the east also. The link between obesity and GERD has been confirmed by various studies. El-Serag and others interviewed 453 hospital employees, and found that 26% had weekly heartburn or regurgitation symptoms.[39] A relationship between obesity and GERD has been seen in Asia. Kang and others studied 2,457 subjects who underwent upper endoscopy in Korea. They found a relationship between higher strata of BMI and presence of erosive esophagitis.[40] Abdominal obesity likely increased intra-abdominal pressure due to transmission of gravitational force of the adipose tissue to the abdominal cavity. Lambert et al. studied morbidly obese patients with a urinary catheter as a surrogate for intra-abdominal pressure, and found that obese patients compare to nonobese patients have higher intra-abdominal pressure.[41,42] This relationship between obesity and intra-abdominal/intragastric pressures has been confirmed by others with use of intragastric manometry **(Fig. 31)**.[29,43]

Epidemiologic studies strongly suggest that the prevalence of GERD is increasing and the major contributing factor to this trend is the rising prevalence of obesity.[41]

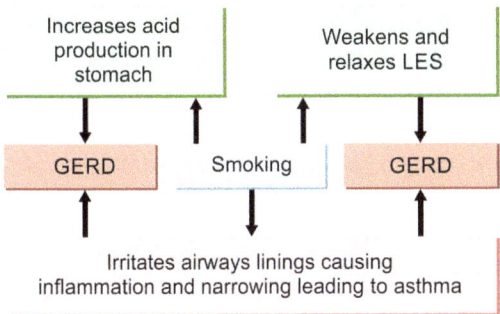

Fig. 29: Smoking causing gastroesophageal reflux disease (GERD) and asthma.

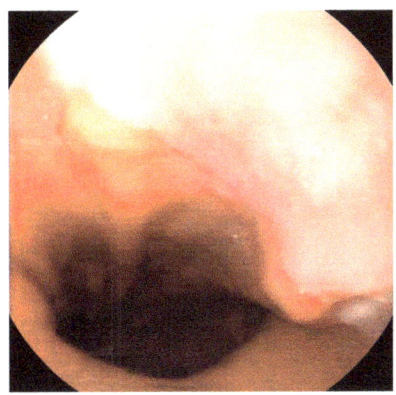

Fig. 30: Gastroesophageal reflux disease (GERD) on endoscopy.

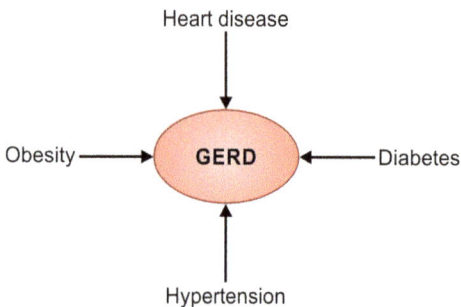

Fig. 31: Comorbidities make gastroesophageal reflux disease (GERD) worse.

In a study by Zhi-Tong Li et al. indicated that GERD patients had significant higher nocturnal BP than non-GERD patients. Antiacid therapy brought about significant reduction in all esophageal monitoring parameters as well as in BP parameters in GERD patients—this study demonstrated that there was significant correlation between hypertension and GERD.

We recommend that all patients of GERD must get proper treatment from an experienced gastroenterologist and if have hypertension then it is more needed. All such patients must reduce weight which has significant positive effect on GERD and hypertension.

Smoking, whether primary or secondary, leads to GERD and asthma-like symptoms. Smoking irritates the mucous lining of airway tubes causing inflammation which leads to edema and thus narrowing of airway tubes. This with thick sticky mucus leads to asthma-like symptoms.

AS IF ASTHMA WAS NOT SUFFICIENT, GASTROESOPHAGEAL REFLUX DISEASE ALSO ATTACKED HIM

Ram was a busy and successful manager in a multinational company. One week before annual reports were due, he came down with a bad flu with severe attack of acidity. He was a known sufferer from bronchial asthma also. The asthma also raised the head and made his condition worst. The attack was so severe that he had to get admitted in a hospital. Though he was suffering with mild acidity, breathlessness, and fatigue for last few years, but this time all the sicknesses attacked him together. He had already tried several medical approaches including homeopathy, conventional medicine, and alternative medicine, but nothing had resolved his problems. The laboratory work revealed that his hematological results were almost within normal range. He was also taking nutritional supplements for long. Now after imaging investigations and upper gastrointestinal endoscopy, doctors at the hospital confirmed that he was suffering with gastroesophageal reflux disease, flu, and bronchial asthma. Though he was not febrile and total leukocyte count was also within normal range, but as a preventive measure physician started salbutamol inhalation along with low dose of steroids. He was put on PPI in morning and evening doses with prokinetic also. His condition improved and he was discharged on 3rd day of admission. At the time of discharge, he was advised to use steroid and salbutamol inhaler for some time, but PPI and prokinetic for 4 weeks and then come for follow-up. He was relieved of his problems and after 4 weeks he was advised to use further 8 weeks PPI and prokinetic (**Figs. 32 and 33**).

Gastroesophageal reflux disease and asthma are from two different organs, esophagus and lungs, but often it is observed that they can occur together. It is not known that what is the cause of their presence simultaneously, but it is known that asthma can worsen GERD if appears in a patient suffering with it. GERD can also worsen asthma (**Figs. 34 and 35**).

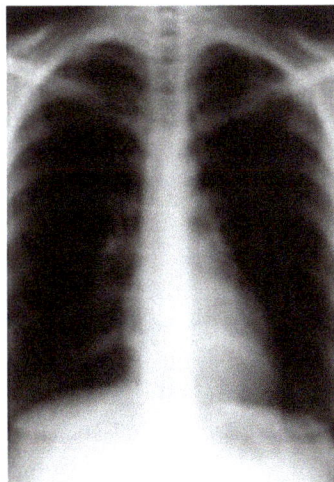

Fig. 32: X-ray chest of Mr Ram.

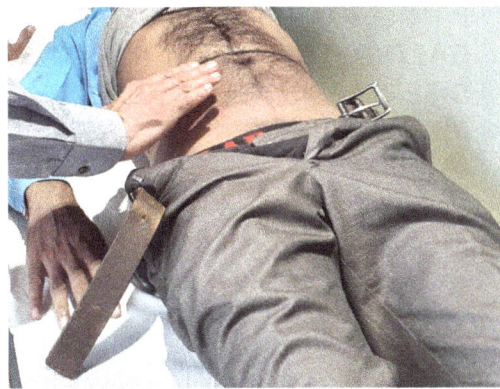

Fig. 34: Patient suffering with gastroesophageal reflux disease (GERD) and asthma.

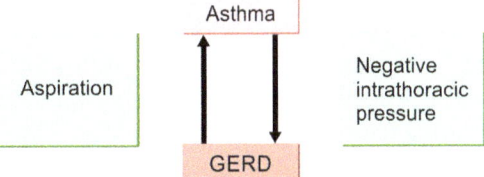

Fig. 35: Interrelation between asthma and gastroesophageal reflux disease (GERD).

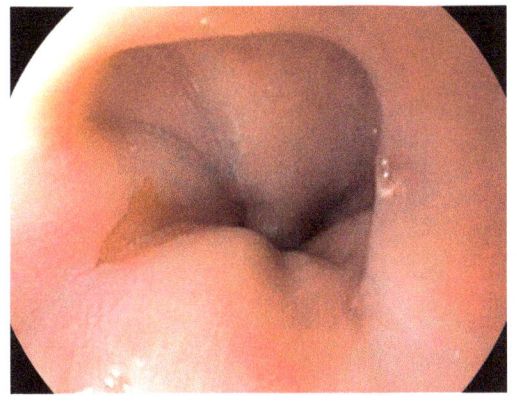

Fig. 33: Gastroesophageal reflux disease (GERD) on endoscopy.

Gastroesophageal reflux disease and asthma can occur in both children and adults. It has been also observed that sometimes GERD can really develop asthma and also it can stimulate the already present asthma making the condition worse. Sometimes incidental aspiration of acid in upper respiratory tract in a chronic case of GERD can cause asthma-like symptoms such as coughing and rarely can lead to pneumonia. It is also noticed by some researchers that in a long-standing cases of GERD laryngeal spasm can happen leading to difficulty in breathing, coughing, and wheezing.

Common extra esophageal manifestations include dental erosion, laryngitis, laryngeal cancer, otitis media, postnasal drip syndrome, sinusitis, cough, hoarseness, chronic obstructive pulmonary disease, recurrent pneumonia, and asthma.[44]

The prevalence of GERD symptoms is often greater in patients with asthma than in general population. In general, some studies have suggested that GERD symptoms such as heartburn and regurgitation are experienced by nearly 80% patients with a diagnosis of asthma.[45]

A study of >100,000 veterans showed that patients with GERD were 1.15 times more likely to have asthma than were those without GERD.[46] In addition, some studies implying pH monitoring have shown a prevalence of GERD of 30–65% among patients with asthma.[47-51]

WHOLE FAMILY SUFFERED WITH GASTROESOPHAGEAL REFLUX DISEASE AND *HELICOBACTER PYLORI* GASTRITIS

Mr Rajat Chopra, a 22-year-old patient, consulted me for heartburn, regurgitation of acid and upper abdominal discomfort and pain with occasional lower chest pain for last 2 years. He was getting relief with antacid gel and cold milk so he was carrying out his life. He, as a young man, was not much worried about his symptoms, but when the chest pain increased in frequency and intensity, he got scared so he came to the hospital with his parents. After examination, he was advised ECG, upper gastrointestinal endoscopy, and ultrasound of abdomen along with routine hematological investigations. Upper gastrointestinal endoscopy revealed that he was suffering with GERD as well as erosive antral gastritis due to *H. pylori*. Urease test was found positive for *H. pylori*. His results of other investigations were within normal range. He was advised morning and evening dose of PPI, algenic acid gel, and a prokinetic for 4 weeks. He was also advised to take care of his drinking water source. Rajat's sickness was explained to his parents and especially about *H. pylori* infection. Next day, his father Mr Rajesh rang me and insisted that he also wants to get his upper gastrointestinal endoscopy done as he was also having similar symptoms as Rajat had. He was having these symptoms longer than his son. His wife Mrs Sheela also told that she was also having similar symptoms, but in a milder form and so she was also not bothered, but after Rajat's diagnosis she was also worried. Probably this family of three persons had gone through about Rajat's problem of GERD and *H. pylori* infection on social media and got information about these problems and so were stressed and scared.

GERD can lead to serious complications and *H. pylori* can cause malignancy if both are not treated and neglected for long.

Mr Rajesh and Mrs Sheela underwent upper gastrointestinal endoscopy next day. Mr Rajesh was having GERD, small hiatus hernia, and antral gastritis. Mrs Sheela was having GERD and antral gastritis. Urease test for *H. pylori* was positive for both Mr Rajesh and Mrs Sheela (**Figs. 36 and 37**).

H. pylori infection can be transmitted to other family members. The estimated prevalence is almost 70% in developing countries, and 30–40% in the United States

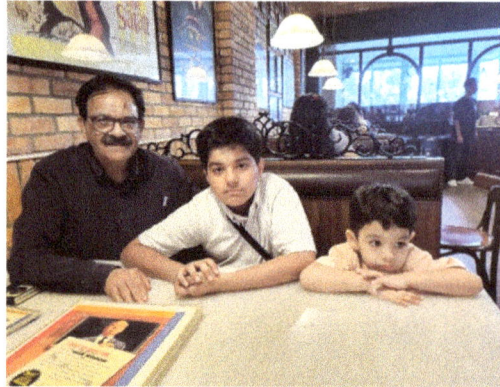

Fig. 36: Whole family can suffer with gastroesophageal reflux disease (GERD) and *H. pylori* infection.

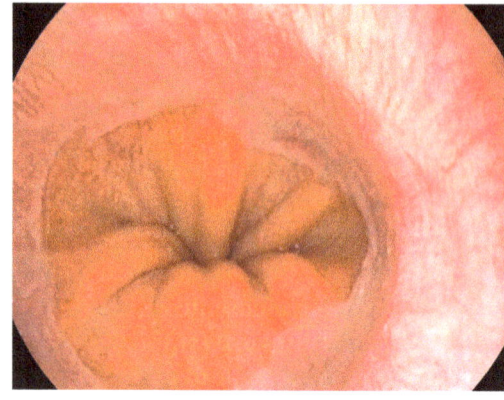

Fig. 37: Gastroesophageal reflux disease (GERD) on endoscopy of Mr Rajat.

and other industrialized countries.[52] In a recent study conducted in Turkey the prevalence of *H. pylori* infection was reported to be 82.5% in the adult population.[53] In developing countries, it is markedly more prevalent at younger ages than it is in developed countries.[54] *H. pylori* infection is high (49.94–83.30%) in India, but the incidence of gastric cancer is comparatively low.....**(Figs. 38 A and B)**.[55]

The most common routes of transmission are fecal-oral and oral-oral routes so it is very common for a family member living together and in an overcrowded situation acquiring *H. pylori* infection easily and so the whole family suffers with *H. pylori* infection and its complications. Children living in such conditions acquire infection of *H. pylori* easily and early than their parents and other adults living in same place. Better hygiene practices and less household overcrowding have contributed to the decline in prevalence over the last decade.[56]

It has been observed that whether a solitary person is suffering with *H. pylori* infection or the whole family suffering with same can be greatly benefited by avoiding contaminated water.

H2-receptor antagonists, proton-pump inhibitors, and antacids are the mainstay of treatment for GERD. *H. pylori* eradication with triple drug therapy gives highly successful results **(Fig. 39)**.

Prokinetics promote the movement of gastrointestinal tract and thus prevent gastric acid stasis and promote gastric emptying of acid and contents **(Fig. 40)**.

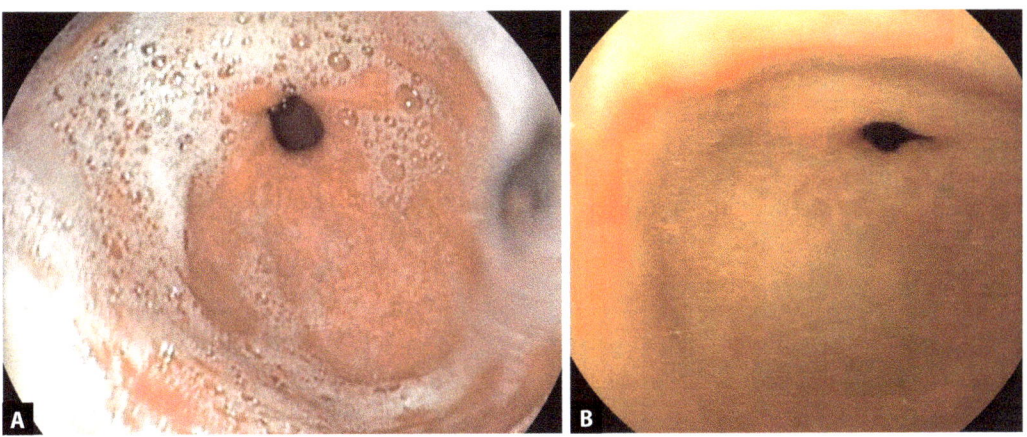

Figs. 38A and B: Erosive antral gastritis, Mr Rajat and Mr Rajesh.

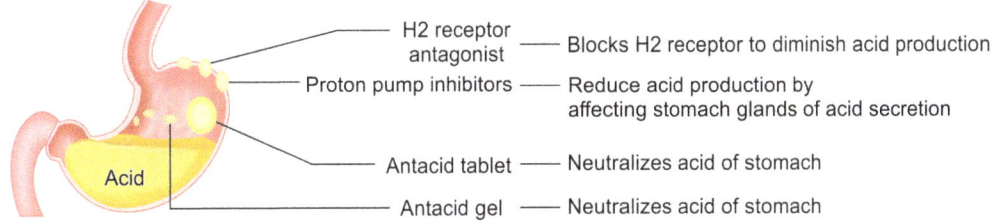

Fig. 39: How antacid, H2-receptor antagonist and proton-pump inhibitors (PPIs) act on stomach acid and its production.

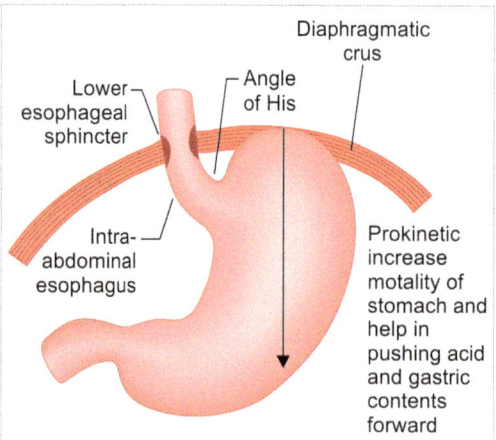

Fig. 40: Mechanism of action of prokinetics.

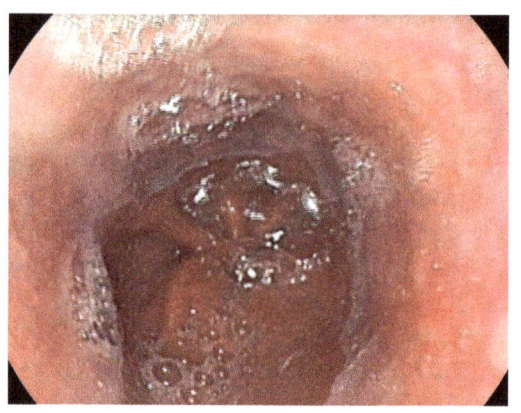

Fig. 41: Early Barrett's esophagus.

NEVER SAY TOO OLD—NO CURE

Mr Ramprasad, aged 82 years, was suffering with heartburn, indigestion, and gas problem for few decades. His problems were not severe and he was not associated with any severe pain though he was having some discomfort and heaviness in upper abdomen, but no pain. He was carrying on his day-to-day work and also working in his tailoring shop regularly from morning till evening. He used to take cold milk and gram sattu for his problem and was also getting relieved. As he was not having any major problem so he was not bothered and did not show to any doctor. He was not much concerned about improving his lifestyle as he was eating whatever was served to him, sometimes skipping breakfast in hurry to go and open his shop. Heartburn, indigestion, and gas problem became usual features for him.

Once he felt chocking sensation in his chest and felt that food was stuck in his upper chest which was relieved after drinking a glass of cold milk. He decided to go to a doctor soon. Few days passed away without showing to any doctor. Again, he developed same attack of chocking sensation and stucking of food in his chest. This time he told his son and went to see a doctor, a private practitioner. The doctor advised him to take some medicines and show to a specialist. When he went to the specialist, he was advised few tests including X-ray of chest, ECG, and upper gastrointestinal endoscopy. X-ray of chest and ECG were within normal range, but upper gastrointestinal endoscopy revealed GERD and early Barrett's esophagus which was diagnosed by histopathology of the biopsied material from the lining of his lower esophagus. He was then explained by the specialist that now you have to take care of your health seriously as Barrett's esophagus may convert to cancer. Mr Ramprasad got scared by listening term "cancer". He promised to the doctor as well as himself that he will follow the advice and treatment given by the doctor. He was also advised to get upper gastrointestinal endoscopy few times at intervals to follow up condition of Barrett's esophagus, improving, or deteriorating. He was also tested by urease test for *H. pylori* which was strongly positive (**Figs. 41 and 42**).

He was advised certain lifestyle changes and PPI and prokinetic. PPI were advised for straight 8 weeks in morning and evening doses and prokinetic once a day. He was also advised alginic acid-based antacid.

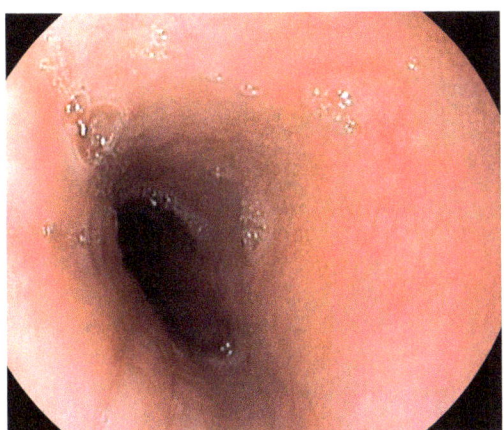

Fig. 42: Barrett's esophagus 1 year after treatment.

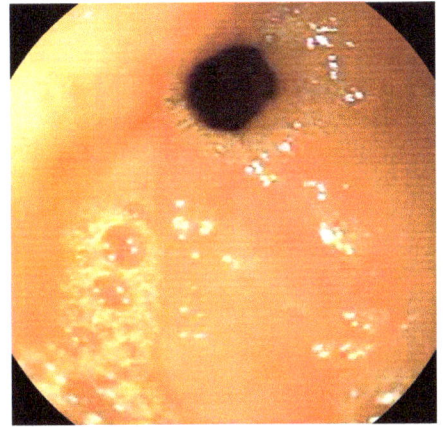

Fig. 43: Erosive antral gastritis due to *H. pylori* infection, on endoscopy.

The lifestyle changes were as avoid alcohol and smoking, eat smaller meals six times a day instead of three big meals, do not lie down for 2–3 hours after a meal, try to maintain weight, while sleeping raise head end of the bed by 8–9 inches, avoid trigger foods which stimulate and increase symptoms, avoid fatty and spicy food, eat multigrain chapatti, and fruits and salads.

Mr Ramprasad was scared to death so he followed doctor's instructions and treatment religiously. He had undergone upper gastrointestinal endoscopy few times and was ultimately told that he is much better. His healing is good. He did not require upper gastrointestinal endoscopy every 3 months, but once a year for one time and if his improvement continued as it was then he will require upper gastrointestinal endoscopy only once in 3 years **(Figs. 43 and 44)**.

Epidemiological and clinical studies suggest that with the advancing age there is an increase in both the prevalence and severity of upper gastrointestinal diseases.[57,58] Gastric acid secretion does not decrease with age, although factors leading to atrophic gastritis, such as *H. pylori* infection, reduce gastric acid secretion.[59] Epidemiological data do not seem to support a role for *H. pylori* in the

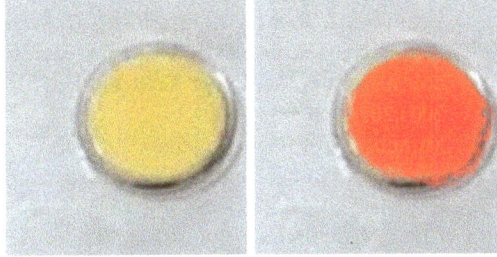

Fig. 44: Rapid urease test—positive, color has changed from yellow to red after placing scrapping from antral area of stomach.

pathogenesis of reflux disease, and suggest a negative association with the increasing incidence of esophageal diseases.[60,61] However, *H. pylori* should be considered in older patients affected by GERD and receiving long-term maintenance treatment with proton-pump inhibitors (PPIs).[62]

Rapid Urease Test

A biopsy of gastric tissue is placed into a medium containing urea and pH indicator. When the bacterial urease splits the urea, the liberated ammonia will increase the pH; this is recognized by a color change in the test indicator. Rapid urease tests are fast, inexpensive, and easy to perform.[63]

REFERENCES

1. Ranjbar R, Khamesipour E, Jonaidi-Jafri N, Rahimi E. Helicobacter pylori in bottled mineral water: genotyping and antimicrobial resistance properties. BMC Microbiol. 2016;16:40.
2. Bahrami AR, Rahimi E, Ghasemian SH. Detection of Helicobacter pylori in City Water, Dental Units' Water, and Bottled Mineral Water in Isfahan. Iran. Sci World J. 2013;2013:280510.
3. Momtaz H, Dehkordi FS, Rahimi E, Asgarifar A. Detection of Escherichia coli, Salmonella species, and Vibrio cholera in tap water and bottled drinking water in Isfahan, Iran. BMC Public Health. 2013;7(13):556.
4. Role-Kampczyk UE, Fritz GJ, Diez U, Lehmann I, Richter M, Herbarth O. Well water-one source of Helicobacter pylori colonization. Int J Hyg Environ Health. 2004;207(4):363-8.
5. Mohebtash M. Helicobacter pylori and its effects on human health and disease. Arch Iran Med. 2011;14(3):192.
6. CDC. Helicobacter Pylori Fact Sheet for Health Care Providers. CDC Stacks. 1998.
7. Ra A, Tobe SW. Acute interstitial nephritis due to pantoprazole. Anns Pharmacother. 2004;38(1):41-5.
8. Calam J, Baron J. ABC of the upper gastrointestinal tract: pathophysiology of duodenal and gastric ulcer and gastric cancer. Br Med J. 2001;323(7319):980.
9. Olbe L, Fandriks L, Hamlet A, Svennerholm AM, Thoreson AC. Mechanisms involved in Helicobacter pylori induced duodenal ulcer disease: an overview. World J Gastroenterol. 2000;6(5):619.
10. Thorell K, Lehours P, Vale FF. Genomics of Helicobacter pylori. Helicobacter. 2017;22:e12409.
11. Camilo V, Sugiyama T, Touati E. Pathogenesis of Helicobacter pylori infection. Helicobacter. 2017;22:e12405.
12. Mobley HL, Mendz GL, Hazell SL. Helicobacter pylori. Helicobacter pylori: Physiology and Genetics. United States: ASM Press; 2001.
13. Serena S, Michele R, Chiara M, Gioacchino L, Lorella F, Tizina M, et al. Relationship between Helicobacter pylori infection and GERD. Acta Biomed. 2018;89(suppl 8):40-3.
14. Slaughter JL, Stenger MR, Reagan PB, Jadcherla SR. Neonatal histamine-2 receptor antagonist and proton pump inhibitor treatment at United States Children's Hospitals. J Pediatr. 2016;174:63-70.
15. Malcolm WF, Cotton CM. Metoclopramide, H2 blockers, and proton pump inhibitors: pharmacotherapy for gastroesophageal reflux in neonates. Clin Perinato, 2012;39(1):99-109.
16. Dilen da Silva CE, Niedermeier BT, Portinho F. Reflux Laryngitis: Correlation between the Symptoms Findings and Indirect Laryngoscopy. Int Arch Otorhinolaryngol. 2015;19(3):234-7.
17. Koufman JA, Aviv JE, Casiano RR, Shaw GY. Laryngopharyngeal reflux: position statement of the committee on speech, voice and swallowing disorders of the American Academy of Otolaryngology-Head and Neck Surgery. Otolaryngol Head Neck Surg. 2002;127(1):32-5.
18. Wang L, Liu X, Liu YL, Zeng FF, Wu T, Yang CL, et al. Correlation of pepsin-measured laryngopharyngeal reflux disease with symptoms and signs. Otolaryngol Head Neck Surg. 2010;143(6):765-71.
19. Koufman JA, Cummins MM. The prevalence and spectrum of reflux in laryngology: a prospective study of 132 consecutive patients with laryngeal and voice disorders. Naples, FL: American Laryngological, Rhinological, and Otological Society, Inc.; 1994.
20. Eckley CA, Rios LdaS, Rizzo LV. Salivary egf concentration in adults with reflux chronic laryngitis before and after treatment: preliminary results. Braz J Otorhinolaryngol. 2007;73(2):156-60.
21. Kahrilas PJ. The role of hiatus hernia in GERD. Yale J Biol Med.1999;72(2-3):101-11.
22. Barham CP, Gotley DC, Alderson D. Precipitating causes of acid reflux episodes in ambulant patients with gastroesophageal reflux disease. Gut. 1995;36:505-10.

23. Michelson E, Siegel CI. The role of the phrenico-esophageal ligament in the lower esophageal sphincter. Surg Gynecol Obstet. 1964;118:1291-4.
24. Torresan F, Mandolesi D, Loannou A, Nicoletti S, Eusebi LH, Bazzoli F. A new mechanism of gastroesophageal reflux in hiatal hernia documented by high resolution impedance manometry: a case report. Ann Gastroenterol. 2016;29(4):548-50.
25. Gordon C, Kang JY, Neild PJ, Maxwell JD. The role of the hiatus hernia in gastroesophageal reflux disease. Aliment Pharmacol Ther. 2004;20:719-32.
26. Modiano N, Gerson LB. Berrett's esophagus: Incidence, etiology, pathophysiology, prevention and treatment. Ther Clin Risk Manag. 2007;3(6):1035-145.
27. Lagergren J, Bergström R, Lindgren A, Nyrén O. Symptomatic gastroesophageal reflux as a risk factor for esophageal adenocarcinoma. N Engl J Med. 1999;340(11):825-31.
28. Mercer CD, Wren SF, DaCosta LR, Beck IT. Lower esophageal sphincter pressure and gastroesophageal pressure gradients in excessively obese patients. J Med. 1987;18:135-46.
29. El-Serag HB, Tran T, Richardson P, Ergun G. Anthropometric correlates of intragastric pressure. Scand J Gastroenterol. 2006;41:887-91.
30. Pandolfino JE, El-Serag HB, Zhang Q, Shah N, Ghosh SK, Kahrilas PJ. Obesity: a challenge to esophagogastric junction integrity. Gastroenterology. 2006;130:639-49.
31. De Luca L, Di Giorgio P, Signoriello G, Sorrentino E, Rivellini G, D' Amore E, et al. Relationship between hiatus hernia and inguinal hernia. Dig Dis Sci. 2004;49(2):243-7.
32. Menon S, Trudgill N. Risk factors in the aetiology of hiatus hernia: a meta-analysis. Eur J. Gastroenterol Hepatol. 2011;23(2):133-8.
33. Franchi M, Ghezzi F, Buttarilli M, Tateo S, Balestreri D, Bolis P. Incisional hernia in a gynecologic oncology, patients: a 10-year study Obstet Gynecol. 2001;97(5P+1):696-700.
34. Leggett CL, Gorospe EC, Calvin AD, Harmsen WS, Zinsmeister AR, Caples S, et al. Obstructive sleep apnea is a risk factor for Barrett's esophagus. Clin Gastroentrol Hepatol. 2014;12(4):583-8.el.
35. de Oliveira SS, dos Santos Ida S, da Silva JF, Machado EC. Gastroesophageal reflux disease: prevalence and associated factors. Arq Gastroenterol. 2005;42(2):116-21.
36. Avidan B, Sonnenberg A, Schell TG, Sontag SJ. No association between gallstones and gastroesophageal reflux disease. Am J Gastroenterol. 2001;96:2858-62.
37. Martinez de Pancorbo C, Carballo F, Horcajo P, Aldeguer M, Villa I, Nieto E. Prevalence and associated factors for gallstone disease: results of a population surgery in Spain. J Clin Epidemiol. 1997;50:1347-55.
38. Rubes AAS, Eduardo MHP, Sergio S, Francisco CBC, Seguro ETB, Ivan C. Prevalence of gallstones in 1,229 patients submitted to surgical laparoscopic treatment of GERD and esophageal achalasia: associated cholecystectomy was a safe procedure. Arq Bras Cir Dig. 2015;28(2):113-6.
39. El-Serag HB, Graham DY, Satia JA, Rabeneck L. Obesity is an independent risk factor for GERD symptoms and erosive esophagitis. Am J Gastroenterol. 2005;100(6):1243-50.
40. Kang MS, Park DI, Oh SY, Yoo TW, Ryu SH, Park JH, et al. Abdominal obesity is an independent risk factor for erosive esophagitis in a Korean population. J Gastroenterol Hepatol. 2007;22(10):1656-61.
41. Paul C, Frank F. Obesity and GERD. Gastroenterol Clin North Am. 2014;43(1):161-73.
42. Lambert DM, Marceau S, Forse RA. Intra-abdominal pressure in the morbidly obese. Obes Surg. 2005;15(9):1225-32.
43. Varela JE, Hinojosa M, Nguyen N. Correlations between intra-abdominal pressure and obesity-related co-morbidities. Surg Obes Relat Dis. 2009;5(5):524-8.
44. Fehmi A, Michael FV. Insite Into the Relationship Between Gastroesophageal Reflux Disease and Asthma. Gastroenterol Hepatol (NY). 2014;10(11):729-36.
45. Field SK, Underwood M, Brant R, Cowie RL. Prevalence of gastroesophageal reflux symptoms in asthma. Chest. 1996;109(2):316-22.

46. El-Serag HB, Sonnenberg A. Comorbid occurrence of laryngeal or pulmonary disease with esophagitis in United States military veterans. Gastroenterology. 1997; 113(3):755-60.
47. American Lung Association Asthma Clinical Research Centers; Mastronarde JG, Anthonisen NR, Castro M, Holbrook JT, Leone FT, et al. Efficacy of esomeprazole for treatment of poorly controlled asthma. N Engl J Med. 2009;360(15):1487-99.
48. Leggett JJ, Johnston BT, Mills M, Gamble J, Heaney LG. Prevalence of gastroesophageal reflux in difficult asthma: relationship to asthma outcome. Chest. 2005;127(4): 1227-31.
49. Kiljander TO, Laitinen JO. The prevalence of gastroesophageal reflux disease in adult asthmatics. Chest. 2004;126(5):1490-4.
50. Harding SM, Guzzo MR, Richter JE. 24-h esophageal pH testing in asthmatics: respiratory symptom correlation with esophageal acid events. Chest. 1999;115(3):654-9.
51. Sontag SJ, O'Connell S, Khandelwal S, Miller T, Nemchausky B, Schnell TG, et al. Most asthmatics have gastroesophageal reflux with or without bronchodilator therapy. Gastroenterology. 1990;99(3):613-20.
52. Barzilay EJ, Fagan RP. Helicobacter pylori. In: Brunette GW (Ed). CDC Health Information for International Travel 2014: The Yellow Book (CDC Health Information for International Travel: The Yellow Book). New York: Oxford University Press; 2014. pp. 80-1.
53. Ozaydin N, Turkyilmaz SA, Cali S. Prevalence and risk factors of helicobacter pylori in Turkey: a nationally-representative, cross-sectional, screening with 13C-Urea breath test. BMC Public Health. 2013;13:1215.
54. World Gastroenterology Organization. World Gastroenterology Organization Global Guideline: Helicobacter pylori in developing countries. J Clin Gastroenterol. 2011;45(5):383-8.
55. Misra V, Pandey R, Misra SP, Dwivedi M. Helicobacter pylori and gastric cancer: Indian enigma. World J. Gastroenterol. 2014;20(6):1503-9.
56. Eusebi LH, Zagari RM, Bazzoli F. Epidemiology of Helicobacter pylori infection. Helicobacter. 2014;19 Suppl. 1:1-5.
57. Pilotto A, Franceschi M. Helicobactor pylori infection in older people. World J Gastroenterol. 2014;20(21):6364-73.
58. Pilotto A, Franceschi M. Upper Gastro-intestinal Disorders. In: Halter JB, Ouslander JG, Tinetti ME (eds). Hazzard's Geriatric Medicine and Gerontology, 6th edition. United States of America: The McGraw-Hill Companies Inc; 2009. pp. 1075-90.
59. Hurwitz A, Brady DA, Schaal SE, Samloff IM, Dedon J, Ruhl CE. Gastric acidity in older adults. JAMA. 1997;278:659-62.
60. Sharma P, Vakil N. review article: Helicobacter pylori and reflux disease. Aliment Pharmacol Ther. 2003;17:297-305.
61. Corley DA, Kubo A, Levin TR, Block G, Habel L, Rumore G, et al. Helicobacter pylori and gastroesophageal reflux disease: a case-control study. Helicobacter. 2008;13: 352-60.
62. Pilotto A, Malfertheiner P. Review article: an approach to Helicobacter pylori infection in the elderly. Aliment Pharmacol Ther. 2002;16:683-91.
63. Nurgalieva ZZ, Goodman KJ, Graham DY. Helicobacter pylori, Encyclopedia of Gastroenterology. 2004;pp. 272-279.

Abbreviations

Life is really simple, but we as humans make it complicated.
–Unknown

BE: Barrett's esophagus
BMI: Body mass index
CNS: Central nervous system
Dx: Diagnosis
DDx: Differential diagnosis
FDA: Food and Drug administration
GEJ: Gastroesophageal junction
GER: Gastroesophageal reflux
GERD: Gastroesophageal reflux disease
GI: Gastrointestinal
GTT: Glucose tolerance test
GU: Genitourinary
Gyn: Gynaecology
HRQL: Health-related quality of life
HH: Hiatus hernia
H2R: H_2-Receptor

H2RA: H_2-receptor antagonist
LES: Lower esophageal sphincter
LESRs: Lower esophageal sphincter relaxations
LESR: Lower esophageal sphincter relaxation
MRI: Magnetic resonance imaging
NSAID: Nonsteroidal anti-inflammatory drugs
NG: Nasogastric
OTC: Over-the-counter
PPI: Proton pump inhibitor
PUD: Peptic ulcer disease
QoL: Quality of Life
RF: Radiofrequency
SCJ: Squamocolumnar junction
TLESR: Transient lower esophageal sphincter relaxations
UES: Upper esophageal sphincter
UGI: Upper gastrointestinal

Multiple Choice Questions and True/False

Nothing in this World is complicated, only misunderstood.
–Chloe Gong

Multiple Choice Questions

Q.1. People suffering with gastroesophageal reflux disease (GERD) should avoid foods and drink.

a. Mint, tomatoes   b. Caffeine, alcohol
c. Vinegar   d. All the above

Ans. d

Q.2. Reflux is an alternative term for:

a. Salivation
b. Acid erosion
c. Nausea and vomiting
d. Regurgitation

Ans. d

True or False

Q.1. Once on a proton pump inhibitor (PPI), always on a PPI.

False

Q.2. If you have heartburn, you have GERD.

False

Q.3. You can take over-the-counter (OTC) medicines without physician's advice.

False

Q.4. If you undergo surgery for GERD, you will not be able to eat normally again.

False

Q.5. GERD is the back up of stomach acid into the esophagus.

True. Acid with gastric contents goes back into esophagus.

Q.6. Babies and children do not develop GERD.

False. People of all ages can suffer from GERD.

Q.7. Reflux is an alternative term for regurgitation.

True. Regurgitation means backward flow.

Q.8. GERD can be diagnosed by blood tests.

False. GERD is diagnosed by trial PPI treatment and endoscopy.

Q.9. Barrett's esophagus (BE) is a serious problem (complication) of GERD.

True. BE becomes precancerous and even turns into cancer.

Q.10. GERD does not affect quality of life.

False. GERD affects the physical as well as mental health of an individual negatively affecting quality of life.

Q.11. Excessive acid production in stomach causes GERD.

False. It is due to moving backward of acid with gastric content into esophagus from stomach.

Q.12. GERD complications affect only esophagus.

False. GERD can also cause asthma, laryngitis, dental enamel erosion, and stomatitis.

Q.13. Stress can cause GERD.

True. Stress can influence the symptoms of GERD. It can worsen the suffering.

Q.14. There is no proper treatment or cure for GERD.

False. There are several management ways for GERD, both medical and surgical.

Q.15. GERD cannot cause serious problem or complications.

False. If GERD is not properly treated, it can cause erosions, strictures, and Barrett's esophagus.

Q.16. Heartburn can cause heart problems.

False. There is no relation between heartburn and heart disease.

Q.17. Drinking cold milk can treat GERD.

False. Milk can neutralize acid initially but then it stimulates more acid production.

Q.18. Poor diet is the cause of heartburn.

False. Diet rich in fatty foods is the cause but there are other causes, the main is reflux of acid and gastric contents into esophagus.

Q.19. Eat before going to bed.

False. Even if you do not eat 2-3 hours before going to bed, it may help, but on lying acid moves up in esophagus from stomach.

Q.20. GERD is an abbreviation or acronym.

Acronym. Abbreviation is a shortened form of a word used in place of full word. An acronym is a word formed for the first letters of each words in a phrase or name.

Index

Page numbers followed by *'f'* figure; and *'t'* indicate table respectively.

A

Abdomen, pain of 34, 39, 55*f*, 57*f* 68, 82, 90
Abdominal esophagus 6, 7
    relations of 8
Abdominal straining 30
Acetylcholine 19*f*, 19
Achalasia 54, 59
Acid
    and food regurgitations 44
    in stomach 16*f*
        causing inflammation 17*f*
    pocket 83
    reflux 95
        crosses 41
        home remedies for immediate relief in 71
    regurgitation 34, 37, 82
        endoscopy 37*f*
    sensitivity 55
    suppression, empirical test of 51
Adenosine 18
Adventitia 24
Alcohol
    consumption, stop 67
    excessive amount of 55
Alginic acid antacids 89
Aloe Vera juice 71
American Academy of Otolaryngology and Head and Neck Surgery 41
Angina pectoris 54, 55
Angle of His
    and gastroesophageal reflux disease 13
    diagrammatic representation of 14*f*
    endoscopic representation of 14*f*
    functions of 13
Antacids 67, 89
    side effects of 68
Antireflux
    barrier 31
    mucosectomy 72, 73, 73*f*, 88
Anxiety 55
Asthma 43, 109*f*, 110, 111*f*
Atrophic changes 86

B

Baclofen 69
Barium esophagogram 71
Barium studies 1
Barium swallow 51
Barrett's esophageal mucosa 77*f*
    on endoscopy 77*f*
Barrett's esophagus 1, 60, 63, 75, 76, 79, 79*f*, 92, 103, 104, 105*f*, 114*f*, 115*f*, 119
    causing 50
    diagnosis 76
    dysplasia in 78
    endoscopic surveillance for 79
    in gastroesophageal reflux disease 76
    management of 78
    pathogenesis of 76
    per prague classification of 76, 77*f*, 77
Belching 40
    repeated 34
Beta-adrenergic agonists 18
Biliary reflux 108*f*
Blood in vomit 4
Body mass index 28, 119
Bowel, herniated loops of 106*f*
Breath, bad 42
Burning sensation 60

C

Caffeine, excessive amount of 55
Calcium
    gene-related peptide 18
    inflex, suppression of 19
Cancer
    develop 76, 79, 92
    early 79
    esophageal 60, 79, 92
    incidence 78
Cardiac pain, usual 39
Central nervous system 119
Cervical esophagus 6, 7
    on cross-section 8*f*
    veins 11
Chemical
    accidental swallowing of 60
    clearance 20
Chest, fire in 3
Chest pain 34, 38*f*, 38, 39, 44, 55, 63, 82
    in gastroesophageal reflux disease 39
    noncardiac 38, 43
Chest pain syndromes 11
Chewing gum 71
Choking 60
Cholecystectomy, laparoscopic 108*f*
Cholecystokinin 18
Cholelithiasis 54, 56
    chronic 107
Cholinergic drugs 19
Cimetidine 68, 89
Circular layer, internal 24
Cisapride 69, 90
Citrus fruits 56
Collar sling fibers 13
Columnar epithelium 75
Columnar-lined esophagus 75
Constrictor muscle, inferior 16
Corkscrew esophagus 21
Coronary veins 11
Cough 34
    chronic 43
    in gastroesophageal reflux disease 41
Cricopharyngeus 16
Crural diaphragm 31
Cryoablation 78

D

Deep abdominal breathing 95
    technique of 93
Depression 90
Dexlansoprazole 69
Diaphragm
    contraction of 41
    right crus of 10
Diaphragmatic crura 10
Diarrhea 90

Diet, six-food elimination 65
Disease, course of 44
Domperidone 69, 90
Dopamine 18
Drowsiness 90
Duodenal ulcer 98
Duodenitis 55
Dysphagia 40, 44, 60, 63, 82
    guidelines in high-grade 75

E

Electrocardiogram 103
Endoabdominal
    subdiaphragmatic 10
Endoscopy 33, 99*f*-103*f*, 108*f*, 109, 111, 115
    esophageal biopsy 50, 51, 52, 78
    stomach in 85*f*
    upper gastrointestinal 1, 40, 50, 52, 55*f*, 84
    role of 44
Endothoracic 10
Eosinophilic esophagitis 60, 63
    mild, severe 64*f*
Erosive antral gastritis 98*f*, 113*f*, 115*f*
Eructation 40
Escherichia coli 98
Esomeprazole 69
Esophageal
    acid clearance acts 19
    adenocarcinoma 60
    biopsy 33
    carcinoma 63
    impedance 51, 52
    manometry 50, 51, 71
    mucosa 21, 32
        acid injury, healing of 71
        mucus covering of 21
        normal 77*f*
        on endoscopy normal 77*f*
        resistances 21
    peristalsis 17, 17*f*
        primary 17
    pH testing 71
    shortening 30
    sphincter 101
    stricture 60, 63, 92
        symptoms of 60
    varices
        early 13*f*
        site of 13*f*
Esophagectomy 79
Esophagitis 63, 92
    drug-induced 63, 65
    healing rates of 68
    Los Angeles classification of 45, 45*f*, 46*f*
    mild 64*f*
    severe 64*f*
Esophagogram 51
Esophagus 8*f*, 16, 100*f*, 106*f*
    adenocarcinoma of 78
    anatomy of 5
    and respiratory system, development of 5*f*
    blood supply of 11, 11*f*
    cancer of 60
    histology of 23
    in relation to right and left crura of diaphragm 8*f*
    lower end of 13*f*
    lymphatic drainage of 11
    mucosa of 21, 23
    nerve supply of 12, 14*f*
    normal 79*f*
        mucosa of 24*f*
    parts of 6
    physiology of 16
    rings of 40*f*
    structure of 23*f*
    surgical anatomy of 5
    thoracic and abdominal parts of 8*f*
    transmits 16
    venous drainage of 11, 12*f*
    vertebral column in normal 7*f*

F

Famotidine 68, 89
Fatty diet 30
Food
    bolus, movement of 17*f*
    caught in throat, feeling of 44
    cause heartburn 93
    fatty 32, 56
    fried 56
    impaction in chest, feeling of 63
    over esophagus 94
    spicy 32, 56
    swallowing of solid 40
    to avoid 93*f*
    to take 93*f*

G

Gallbladder 108*f*
Gallstones 54, 56, 57*f*, 107, 107*t*
Gas problem 34
Gastric arteries 11
Gastric atrophy 86
Gastric mucosal folds 83
Gastritis 55, 99*f*
    chronic 54, 57
    endoscopic view of 58*f*
    erosive 54*f*
Gastroesophageal junction 8, 10*f*, 16, 31, 119
    intrinsic or internal 9*f*
    surgical anatomy of 5
Gastroesophageal reflux disease 1, 2, 3*f*, 28, 29, 31, 38*f*, 39*f*, 41*f*, 54*f*, 58*f*, 60, 63, 66, 70, 91, 92*f*, 97, 97*f*, 99, 100, 100*f*, 101, 101*f*, 102, 102*f*, 103, 104, 105*f*, 106*f*, 107, 108, 108*f*, 109*f*, 110, 110*f*, 111, 111*f*, 112, 112*f*, 119
    affect quality of life 92
    ageing 32
    and infants 29
    chronic
        drug therapy for 70
        symptoms of 44
    classic symptoms of 34, 34*t*, 39, 50
    clinical features of 34
    complications of 63
    dangerous 91
    diagnosis of 50, 54, 91
    different conditions mimicking 54
    early 26*f*
    endoscopic
        treatment procedures for 72
        view of 58*f*
    epidemiology of 26, 27
    etiology of 28
    extraesophageal symptoms of 43*f*, 43
    global distribution of 26*f*
    heartburn of 35*f*
    history of 75
    incidence of 26, 88
    incompetent 3*f*
    increase symptoms of 95
    lower esophageal sphincter causing 30
    management of 67
    medical treatment, failure of 69
    mild 52*f*
    morbidity and mortality 27

nonspecific treatment of 70
overeating 31
pain in epigastrium in 3
pathophysiology of 31
pharmacology of drugs used in 89
prevalence of 26
prognosis 66
recent advancements and modern trends in 88
risk of 20*t*, 28, 31, 95
severe 52*f*
site of pain in abdomen in 57*f*
sore throat in 41, 41*f*
step-up and step-down treatment 70
suffering 91, 92
surgical treatment of 71
symptoms of 34
tests to diagnose 51
treatment of 67
trigger foods 32, 32*f*
types or grades of 96
with abdomen pain 39*f*
with chest pain 38*f*
Gastrointestinal bleeding 63
Gastrointestinal smooth muscle 9
Gastroparesis 61
Ginger 71
Gingivitis 34, 43
Gingivitis, oral cavity for 50
Globus sensation 43
Glossitis 34, 43, 50
Glucose tolerance test 119
Gut bacteria 2
Gut brain disorder 55
Gut mucosal inflammation 2

H

H_2-receptor antagonist 89
   side effects of 89
Halitosis 34, 42, 89
Health-related quality of life 119
Healthy weight, maintain 67
Heartburn 3, 34, 35, 44, 63
   burning feeling of 36
   causes of 82, 92, 94, 94*f*
   factors of 93*f*
   lifestyle problem 93
   smoking cause 94
Helicobacter pylori 57, 85, 98
   antral gastritis 85*f*
   bacteria in stomach 86*f*
   bacterium 86*f*
   gastritis 50, 57, 99, 112
   infection 28, 85, 86, 97, 112*f*, 115*f*

Hemorrhage 63
Hernia, umbilical 104, 106, 106*f*
Hiatal hernia 29, 30, 82, 83*f*, 95-119
   and gastroesophageal reflux disease 29
   lifestyle measure 95
   pushes lower esophageal sphincter 83
   type of 83
Hiatus hernia 101*f*, 102, 103, 103*f*, 104, 106*f*
Hiccups 41
Histamine-2 receptor antagonists 68
Hoarseness of voice 44
   to laryngitis 34, 41
Hormonal influence 70
Hydrochloric acid 16, 89, 92
Hypertension 108

I

Indigestion 42
Infectious esophagitis 63, 65
Inflamed esophagus 79*f*
Inflammation 25
Intensive care unit 103
Itopride 69, 90

J

Jackhammer esophagus 20
Jaggery 71
Junction, intrinsic or internal 9

L

Laimer, phrenoesophageal fascia of 10
Lansoprazole 69
Laryngitis 101*f*
   larynx for 50
Laryngoesophageal reflux disease
   cause of 47
   complications of 47
   diagnosis of 47
   symptoms 47
   treatment of 47
Laryngopharyngeal reflux disease 41
Laryngotracheal diverticulum 5
Levosulpiride 90
Lifestyle changes 67, 78
Lifestyle management 47
Los Angeles classification
   advantages of 46

   esophagitis, grades of 45
   limitations of 46
Lower esophageal sphincter 3*f*, 6*f*, 9, 16, 17, 19*f*, 20*f*, 31, 35*f*, 36*f*, 106*f*, 119
   competent 2*f*
   factors weakening 47
   intrinsic component of 10
   overeating putting pressure on 37*f*
   physiology of 18
   relaxation 10, 19, 119
   strong 19*t*
   surgical anatomy of 5
   weak 19*t*
Lymphocytic esophagitis 63, 65

M

Magnetic resonance imaging 119
Malignancy, incidence of development of 75
Medigus ultrasonic surgical endostapler 72, 73*f*, 88
Metaplasia 24
Metoclopramide 69
Milk
   butter 71
   cold 71
Mint 71
Mosapride 69
Mouth 43*f*
   dry 89
Mucosa 23
   heals faster 71
Muscle layer 24
Muscular components 18
Myosin phosphorylation, cessation of 19

N

Nausea 34, 42, 90
   vomiting 34, 42
Neonatal intensive care unit 101
Nicotine 18
Nissen's fundoplication 71
Nitrate 76
Nitric oxide 18, 20*f*
Nizatidine 68, 89
Nonerosive reflux disease 24
Nonsteroidal anti-inflammatory drugs 79, 119
Nonulcer dyspepsia 54, 55
   case of 55*f*
Nose, runny 89
Nutcracker esophagus 20

O

Obesity 28, 32, 108
Odynophagia 40
  pain of 40
Omeprazole 69
Osteoporosis 68
Otolaryangology and head and neck surgery 102
Over-the-counter
  acid reducing medication 26
  analgesics 27
  medicine, off and on reflux symptoms use 1

P

Pain
  in neck 60
  site of 107f
  upper abdomen 39, 39f
Pancreatitis, chronic 61
Pangastric infection leads 86
Pangastritis 100f
Pantoprazole 69
Paraesophageal
  hiatal hernia 82f
  junction, physiology of 18
Peppermint 32
Peptic ulcer disease 50, 54, 54f, 85, 119
Peritoneum 10
pH monitoring 51, 52
Phrenic artery, inferior 11
Phrenic vein, inferior 11
Phrenoesophageal ligament 10, 10f, 31
  acts 10
Phrenoesophageal membrane 9
Pineapple juice 71
Pleura 10
Pneumonitis, recurrent 44
Portocaval anastomosis 13f
Pregnant, treatment of 70
Prepyloric gastritis 99f
Prokinates 69
Prokinetics
  drugs 90
  mechanism of action of 114f
Prostaglandin E 18
Proton pump inhibitor 27, 38, 51, 69, 78, 89, 101, 113f, 119
  side effects of 89
  therapy 66, 78
Protozoan infection 40
Psychological factor 55

Pylori antral gastritis 58f
Pyrosis 44, 50

Q

Quality of life 119

R

Rabeprazole 69
Radiation therapy 60
Radiofrequency 119
Radiofrequency ablation 72, 78, 88
  balloon 72f
Ranitidine 68, 89
Rapid urease test 115, 115f
  positive 58f
Reflux esophagitis 38, 63
Refluxed material per episode, quantity of 42
Renzapride 69
Retroperitoneal veins 11
Rumination syndrome 37

S

Salivation, excessive 44
Salmonella typhimurium 98
Sandifer syndrome 44
Schatzki ring 40
Secretin 18
Skeletal muscle component 18
Skin, dry 89
Sleep disorders 44
Sleeping disturbances 89
Sliding hiatus hernia 82f
Smooth muscle component 18
Splenic veins 11
Squamocolumnar junction 119
Squamous epithelium,
  metaplasia of 75
Stomach
  acid 113f
  herniation of part of 84
  normal 82f, 83f
  pregnant uterus putting pressure on 36f
Stomatitis 34, 43
Stratum corneum 23
Stratum germinativum 24
Stratum spinosum 24
Stress 30, 55
  meditation reduces 94f
Stretta system 72
Submucosa 24
Subpleural fascia 10

Swallowing
  and dysphagia, pain in 34
  difficulty in 4
  painful 4, 40, 63

T

Teeth enamel erosion 34, 42, 42f
Thoracic esophagus 6, 7
Throat 43f
Tinnitus 89
Transient lower esophageal sphincter relaxation 10, 119
Transoral incisionless fundoplication 72, 73f, 88
Transversalis fascia 10
Tulsi leaves 71

U

Ulcers 63
Upper esophageal sphincter 6f, 13, 16, 119
  factor weakening 47
Upper gastrointestinal 119

V

Vagus nerve yoga 92
Vibrio cholera 98
Voice, rest to 41
Volume clearance 20
Vomiting 34, 42, 44, 90

W

Walnuts 56
Water
  brash 38, 44
  drink plenty of 41
Watermelon juice 71
Weight loss 60

X

X-ray chest 111f

Y

Yoghurt 56

Z

Zenker's diverticulum 59, 60
Z-line 24f
Z-line distorted 25f

EU GSPR Authorised Reprsentative
Logos Europe, 9 rue Nicolas Poussin
1700, La Rochelle, France
Phone: +33 (0) 6 67 93 73 78
E-mail: contact@logoseurope.eu

www.ingramcontent.com/pod-product-compliance
Ingram Content Group UK Ltd.
Pitfield, Milton Keynes, MK11 3LW, UK
UKHW050703160426
5217IPUK00041B/1298